Winning over Cancer

Winning Over Cancer

Collection

Winning OVER Cancer

10 FACTS
I Wish I Knew Before Being Diagnosed

Beating Cancer ...
Regaining Lasting Health

PAULA BLACK

Praise for Winning Over Cancer

“Real hope. *This research is exactly what was missing in our past efforts. What an eye opener.* – **Suzy K.**

“Body soul and spirit approach. Excellent and godly must-read.” – **Phil M.**

“Get this book! *Not a fad. A solution. Courageous author. not afraid to uncover truth.”* – **Neal K.**

“Excellent Information. *Highly encouraging for my cancer situation.”* – **Carrie F.**

“I learned truths that no one told me. It’s changing everything.” – **Bernice S.**

"The title says it all. *Winning Over Cancer. Written simple and honest and super informative. Helped me take my first step." –* **Sharon K.**

"Fantastic Book*. Deeply inspirational. We're buying this book to give to our family and friends. Such valuable information." –* **Deb and Cecil M.**

"Logical and very interesting. Even shocking. This exposes the lies." **Bonnie S.**

"Brilliant! *A MUST read for ANYONE with cancer. Love the body soul spirit approach." –* **Christine G.**

"Self-help to cure any disease! *OMG. Full of need-to-know ways to fight cancer. It's not about symptoms anymore."* **Shawna S.**

"This book was ***fascinating, informative, and makes sense****. I've gone through all the traditional poison and hated the effects and was convinced that it just could not be right. This book is a heaven sent. I wish I had this book at the beginning." –* **Mark T.**

"This truth will save your life*! WOC has the potential of saving millions of lives. So grateful for this information." –* **Natalie B.**

"Stop the runaround. *I've been chasing cancer for three years and finally got this book. This book helped me understand why my treatments aren't working. It helped me with my relationship with God too. I'm now doing this right."* – **Steve T.**

"I'm so happy to have the opportunity to read this book! It's an ***answer to my prayers****."* – **Tasha M.**

"Great research tool. *Her method of juicing, eliminating toxins, building up her immune system along with the spiritual part (body-soul-spirit) was excellent. And effective. It worked. She is cancer free for years."* – **Marlene S.**

"I wish I'd had this book long ago*. I've watched so many friends and family die from cancer. All because we were told false "facts" and believed the doctors knew best. Paula is living proof of "what is true."* – **Dan B.**

"I've known Paula and her husband Dale for decades. They practice what they preach. Always have. Paula's amazing testimony is real and has been a powerful blessing to so many people." – **Barb M.**

"An ***excellent book*** *for finding out what cancer is and how to get rid of it. Wow!"* – **Rob E.**

"Loved the book. ***Excellent information.*** *I recommend buying it if you have cancer. It helped me a lot and is a great starting place for understanding what to do next."* – **Janie A.**

"Spectacular!!! *A true story that blew my mind. Monstrous cancer totally eradicated. Well written page turner."* – **Maria J.**

"Excellent book. *I read it in one day as I could not put it down. So good! Once you know the truth, you can't ignore it."* – **Jan B.**

"This book is great, especially if you have a loved one fighting cancer. Thank you, Paula, for giving us such life-changing information. It's thrilling to see someone who was able to get well without the horrible effects of chemotherapy." – **Susan W.**

"This is a wake-up call. *We have a right to understand what cancer is and what's happening in our body and no one told me. The information in* 'Winning Over Cancer' *shocked me and changed everything I was thinking. I'm so grateful for this powerful information."* – **Michelle O.**

"Absolutely amazing book! ***Eye-opening information.*** *Honest and full of deep truths. I am thanking God for bringing this book to me."* – **Jillian R.**

"Love the body, soul and spirit approach*. This book addresses the key issues of a cancer diagnosis. Having this information helps make sense of something that doesn't seem to make any sense. Its helped me so much and I strongly recommend it for anyone who's been diagnosed."* – **Patricia N.**

Winning Over Cancer

This book is based on the author's personal experiences, research, and faith journey. It is intended for informational, educational, and inspirational purposes only.

Neither Black Eagle Publishing LLC nor the author provides medical advice, diagnosis, or treatment. Nothing in this book is intended to prescribe or replace professional medical care, nor should it be interpreted as a recommendation for any specific protocol, supplement, dietary change, or lifestyle practice.

The content presented in this book—including discussions related to body, soul, and spirit, nutrition, detoxification, emotional healing, and spiritual principles—is not intended to substitute for consultation with qualified healthcare professionals.

Readers are strongly encouraged to seek the advice of their physician or other qualified medical providers regarding any questions they may have about a medical condition or treatment plan. Health-related decisions should always be made in partnership with a licensed medical professional.

While the author shares what she personally learned and applied during her own cancer journey; individual results may vary. No guarantees are made regarding outcomes. The author and publisher expressly disclaims any liability for any loss, injury, or damages alleged to be caused, directly or indirectly, by the use or application of the information contained in this book.

By reading this book, you acknowledge that you are responsible for your own health decisions and actions.

BLACK EAGLE
PUBLISHING, LLC

ISBN: 978-1-965343-09-8 (Print)

ISBN: 978-1-965343-10-4 (E-book)

ISBN: 978-1-965343-11-1 (Audiobook)

10 9 8 7 6 5 4 3 2 1

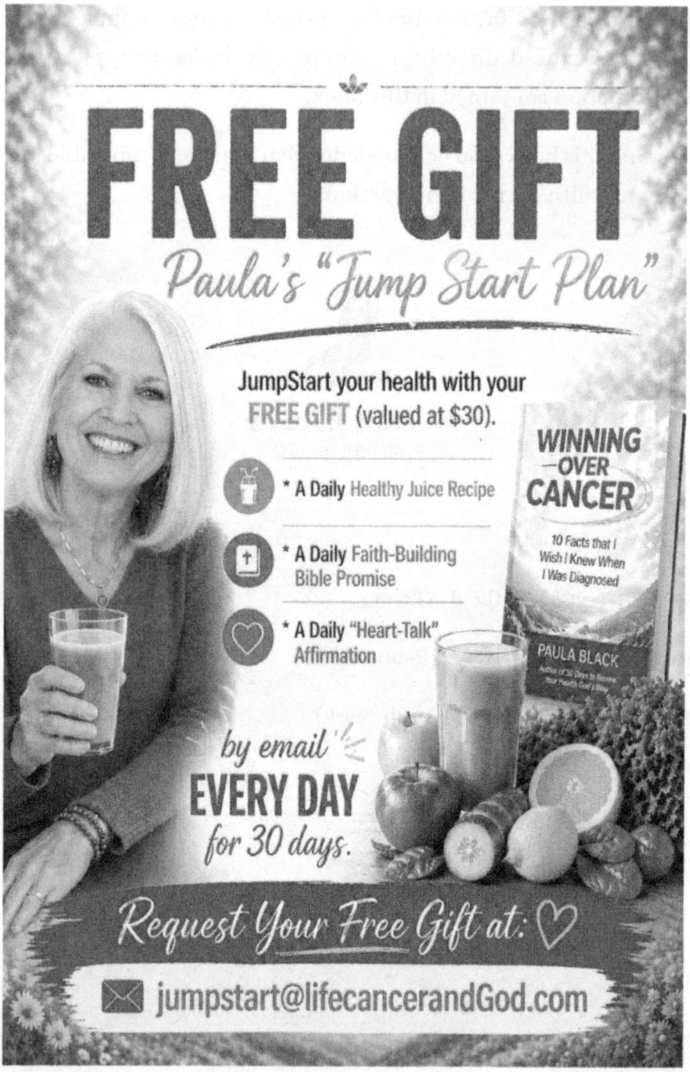
FREE GIFT
Paula's "Jump Start Plan"
JumpStart your health with your
FREE GIFT (valued at $30).
* A Daily Healthy Juice Recipe
* A Daily Faith-Building
Bible Promise
* A Daily "Heart-Talk"
Affirmation
WINNING
OVER
CANCER
10 Facts that I
Wish I Knew When
I Was Diagnosed
PAULA BLACK
by email
EVERY DAY
for 30 days.
Request Your Free Gift at:
jumpstart@lifecancerandGod.com

To my husband, Dale—

From the first moment of diagnosis
to the completion of this book,
you have been my constant—steady in faith,
rich in love, and unwavering in support.
This journey, and this message,
was shaped by your presence
and an invaluable contribution.
With all my love and gratitude.

Disclaimer

The content in this booklet is based on personal experience and research and is provided for informational and inspirational purposes only. It is not intended as medical advice, diagnosis, or treatment.

Readers should consult with licensed healthcare professionals before making changes to their medical care, diet, or lifestyle, especially when dealing with serious conditions such as cancer.

The author does not claim to diagnose, treat, cure, or prevent any disease. Any decisions made based on this content are the sole responsibility of the reader.

Contents

Introduction

Hello, I'm Paula.

If you or someone you love is facing cancer, then you understand how overwhelming and helpless it can feel. Fear, uncertainty, and unanswered questions often surround the journey. Yet in the middle of those difficult moments, there is hope.

One of the greatest struggles many people face is not cancer itself, but a lack of understanding about it. For years, countless families have felt powerless when confronted with disease—believing there were few options beyond prayer and medical treatment. But knowledge brings clarity, and understanding strengthens faith.

The purpose of this book is to offer encouragement, insight, and hope—spiritually, emotionally, and physically. Healing involves more than simply fighting disease; it involves learning how the body was designed to heal, how the mind influences health, and how faith can impact the outcome.

Cancer can leave people feeling afraid, confused, and uncertain about what to do next. Many desperately want to help a loved one heal yet often feel powerless because they don't know where to begin.

One of the most important discoveries on my healing journey was learning that having the right knowledge makes a dramatic difference. Fear often grows where understanding is absent. But wisdom brings clarity, direction, and hope. And as understanding increases, faith becomes stronger and more confident.

The heart behind this book is to encourage and equip those walking through the difficult circumstances of a serious disease. My desire is to offer practical insight and a deeper understanding of how the body, mind, and spirit work together in the healing process.

Looking back at my own journey, there is a deep wish that more had been understood about cancer much earlier in life. When friends and family face the disease, it often seemed that little could be done beyond prayer. At the time, understanding was limited, and where cancer was concerned, faith was weakened by a lack of knowledge.

That reality causes me to think of the Scripture, *"My people are destroyed for lack of knowledge..."* — Hosea 4:6.

At the time of my own diagnosis, I assumed cancer struck at random, without reason or pattern. There were no answers... and therefore, no clear direction.

Those days are far behind me now.

Today, I am much more informed. And it is a joy to share with you some of the truths that brought hope, clarity, and direction along the journey.

This book is not meant to be exhaustive—there are not enough pages in a small book like this to include everything learned over the years. But it *is* a meaningful starting point. In fact, it's the very book I wish someone had placed in my hands the day I was diagnosed.

As you read, please know this: no one is here to judge you, pressure you, or tell you what you should or should not do. My heart is to share—gently, lovingly, and with great respect for wherever you are on your own journey. My prayer is that this information helps you move forward with more confidence and clarity.

A specific moment, a few weeks after the diagnosis, became deeply meaningful. While praying to God with my Bible resting in my lap, this promise from Scripture seemed to stand out with fresh clarity:

"... God is faithful, who will not allow you to be tempted (tested) beyond what you are able, but with the temptation (testing) will also make the way of escape..."
—1 Corinthians 10:13 (author emphasis)

This verse settled deeply into my heart. It reminded me that I was not alone. That God had already made a way forward.

It is my sincere hope that as you read these pages, you will experience peace instead of panic...

Clarity instead of confusion...

Faith instead of fear.

That is what happened to me as I learned the information I am about to share.

In the middle of uncertainty, I chose to seek truth—not opinions, not fear, but truth.

And that truth changed everything.

Because it is *truth* that makes us free (John 8.32).

Paula Black

The question then becomes:
when truth is revealed...
will it be believed?

Chapter 1

It's Cancer

There are moments in life when time doesn't stop...

The room keeps moving.

The clock keeps ticking.

Someone is still talking.

But inside your head, everything goes quiet.

You simply freeze.

I could see the doctor's lips moving. I knew words were coming out. Long words. Medical words. But none of them reached me. It was as if the volume on the entire world had been turned down.

No. I can't hear this.

I can't hear it.

Then one word broke through.

Aggressive.

That word didn't need interpretation.

It didn't need explanation.

It landed like ice water on an already cold day.

They gave the diagnosis an official medical name, something that sounded like Greek to me. I didn't understand it, and I didn't try to. Once you hear the word "*aggressive*," everything else fades into the background noise.

The doctor's recommendation followed quickly.

Another surgery.

Immediately.

To make sure it's all removed.

And I agreed without hesitation.

At the time, I believed cancer was something foreign, a disease inside the body. Something that didn't belong there. Something that had invaded and needed to be removed.

There was only one thought left: shouting.

Get it out of me.

That's what people die from, right? Cancer inside you. So, remove it. Eliminate it. Problem solved.

Looking back now, I realize how common that thinking is. Probably ninety-nine percent of people respond the same way.

Fear simplifies everything. It reduces complex questions to a single desperate command: Get it out.

But that moment... that shock, that instinctive fear, that sudden understanding that life had just shifted without permission... became part of my story.

And then there was my husband, Dale.

He had already watched more than twenty-six close friends and family members lose their lives to cancer.

Twenty-six.

He had stood beside their hospital beds. He had prayed hopeful prayers. He had watched treatments fail. He had attended funerals he never expected to attend.

So, when he heard my diagnosis...

There were no speeches.

No strong declarations.

No instant faith-filled answer.

Just silence.

Because when you've seen cancer take that many people, the word doesn't arrive gently. It doesn't knock politely at the door.

It storms in carrying faces you loved... and memories you wish you didn't have to relive.

In that moment, both of us stood at the edge of the unknown.

I didn't know yet that this diagnosis would not be the end of my story.

I didn't know it would challenge everything I thought I understood about medicine, healing, and God.

I didn't know it would lead me on a journey that would reshape my understanding of fear, belief, and faith.

All I knew was this: Life had changed.

And a new story had begun.

My name is Paula Black. For over two decades, I've been a Faith-Based Wellness Coach and Bible teacher. I'm the creator and teacher of the *Winning Over Cancer Coaching Program.* I'm also co-author of the book *Life, Cancer & God*, my story of how I overcame terminal cancer naturally using a body, soul, and spirit approach —without chemo, radiation, or more surgery.

Since my recovery more than twenty-five years ago, I've heard from countless people who reach out during one of the most frightening moments of their lives.

Often, it's a spouse, a parent, a child, or a close friend of someone who has just received a diagnosis. They usually say the same thing:

"I want to help them... but I don't know where to start. They've been diagnosed with cancer, and I don't know what to do."

Other times, the person contacting me is the one who has just been diagnosed.

If you or someone you love is facing cancer, you're in the right place. This book was written for you. It's a first step, a way to start moving in a good direction, a way to begin taking back control through increased knowledge and understanding.

You may feel frightened right now. You may be

imagining the worst. But you should know something important:

You have time.

You have options.

Right after a diagnosis, the most important step is this: slow down.

Pause. Gather truthful information.

Over the years, I've seen the same mistake again and again.

People rush.

They make life-changing decisions too quickly.

I understand the pressure.

I understand the urgency.

I truly do.

But with over twenty years as a faith-based wellness coach, this is what I've learned... and what I would tell my own family:

Slow down.

Learn.

Become informed.

By the time you finish this book, I believe you will see it clearly:

You do have time.

You do have options.

Chapter 2

What To Do First

What you understand about cancer is important. Because what you do *first* can *greatly* shape everything that follows.

You have space to pause.

And time to educate.

To take your first steps thoughtfully and wisely.

Winning Over Cancer offers grounded information at a time when your world is shaking. This book helps point toward hope rather than fear. Most importantly, it provides solid steppingstones forward—reminding you that you are not powerless, you are not alone, and there is a path to renewed health ahead, one step at a time.

An Unplanned Storm

When I was diagnosed, it felt like a monster storm had come out of nowhere.

In Matthew 7, Jesus speaks about the importance of building your house on the rock. Some build on sand, while others build on solid rock. The difference becomes clear when a storm comes. The storm reveals the strength of the foundation.

And storms *do* come.

When we have a strong foundation *before* the storm arrives, we can stand. But when the storm hits unexpectedly, we often find ourselves trying to build while the wind is already raging.

That's exactly where I found myself. That might describe you as well.

I had to begin building my foundation in the middle of the storm. Even though my own mother, aunt, and grandfather had been previously diagnosed with cancer, I never learned the information that I'll share with you in this book. Had I known these secrets earlier, it would have made a profound difference and impacted many of my early decisions.

To handle the storm of a cancer diagnosis wasn't easy. And it wasn't instant. But I learned to become steady. My knowledge grew as did my faith. Step by step, a plan formed.

And ultimately, my plan worked.

You may be uncertain, overwhelmed, and unsure how to navigate something as frightening and complex as cancer. But your diagnosis does not define the end of your story. There *is* a way forward. Health and healing begin with taking the first step.

What you do first matters. That first step often sets the direction for what follows. It begins to shape the path ahead and sets your sights on a future that may still feel far away.

Despite your first steps, you can always pause and change direction—I did. As I educated myself about cancer, the proposed treatments, and the options before me, what I learned began to shift my thinking—and fairly quickly led me to change course.

Whether you feel prepared for what you are now facing—or not—there is genuine reason to be hopeful. Why? Because you're seeking answers. The very fact that you're reading *Winning Over Cancer* indicates that you are not surrendering to fear or confusion. Instead, you are looking for guidance, clarity, and direction after hearing that you—or someone you love—has been diagnosed with cancer.

There is a lot of valuable information available here —information that will likely change what you know about cancer, and how to rebuild lasting health. By learning simple, natural ways to care for your body and spiritual truths that bring healing, you can begin to feel more confident and hopeful about what lies ahead.

The goal of these pages is to offer understanding in place of the fear that often surrounds the word *cancer*. Together, let's explore what's really happening and what you're *truly* dealing with. As I said in the last chapter, you *do* have options.

This is not the end of your story. What you're learning here may be the very beginning of taking your health back—thoughtfully, wisely, and with the truths needed for a future free from cancer.

It is not my intention to challenge the medical system or standard cancer protocol. My family and I have benefited greatly from medical treatment in previous years. Many of our close friends are doctors, nurses, and healthcare professionals.

I am not a licensed medical professional, and this book does not offer medical advice. Nor does it direct anyone regarding what they should or should not do. Instead, it shares lessons learned and the steps taken throughout my personal healing journey. It also reflects what would have been helpful to know from the beginning and what I wish I'd known on day one, when I was diagnosed.

Although my journey began without the knowledge shared in this book, one thing was done right from the start—my trust was placed in God and His Word. That decision set my course and provided direction to a place of safety, where the truths needed to overcome cancer were revealed.

I now look back with gratitude for the things learned and the personal growth I experienced through the process.

This is only the beginning. The next chapter offers further insight and practical steps to support continued progress—one faithful step at a time.

Someone Have Cancer?

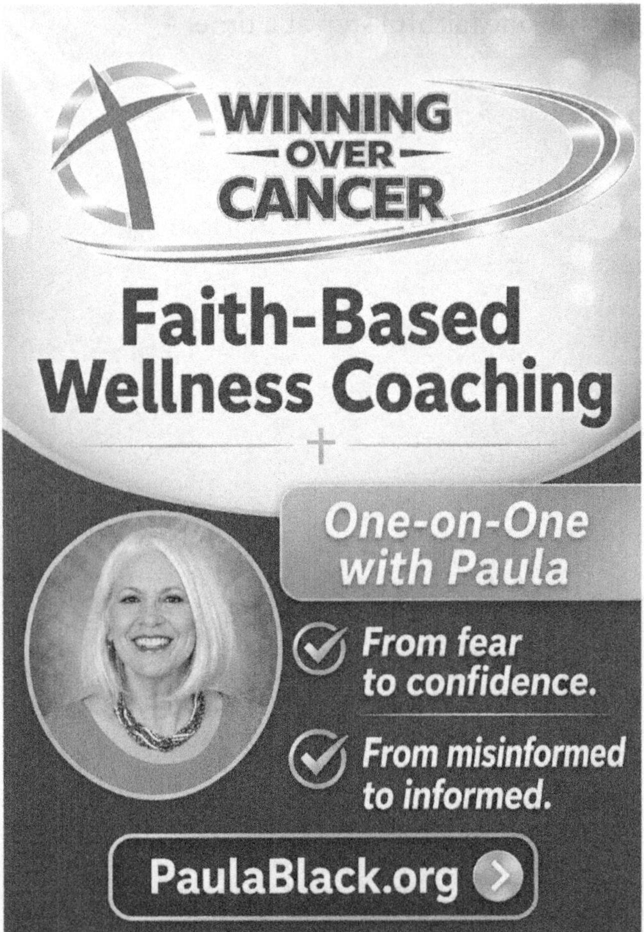

Chapter 3

Hidden in Plain Sight

My early discoveries revealed foundational truths about cancer and healing that changed both my direction and outcome. My entire cancer journey, from diagnosis to restored health, is detailed in my book, *Life, Cancer & God.*

Unlocking those same secrets has helped many others throughout the years. Perhaps they will help you, too.

Educate Yourself

My hope is that the information in *Winning Over Cancer* —along with additional resources and teaching available through PaulaBlack.org—will empower you to make thoughtful, informed choices that lead to restoration and lasting health. *(Additional video teaching and coaching resources are currently in development. Join our email list for updates.)*

Cancer involves life and death. At its core, it follows the law of cause and effect. In my personal journey, cancer developed from the accumulation of choices I made along life's way—some significant, others seemingly small.

After it became clear what cancer is and how it behaves in the body, it was fairly easy to change the circumstances—the *cause*. And reverse my situation—the *effect*.

Yes, it took time and diligence. But that was a small price to pay to become cancer-free.

One of the most important lessons I ever learned came just in the nick of time. I wish it had come sooner. But still, I was grateful to receive it when it finally arrived. It came from a family friend who was a medical doctor. She took me aside and said, "Paula, there's no need to panic, no need to rush ahead in fear. Instead, take time to educate yourself. Take time to learn about cancer and the treatments you're being urged to receive. Take some time to understand your situation clearly. Misinformation is everywhere. Learn the truth. Once you've gained enough understanding about cancer and the treatments being offered, then you can make informed decisions about how to proceed."

She encouraged me to pause, to learn about my condition, to study carefully, and to consider my options prayerfully. Her words carried a deeper lesson—that taking time to become informed is not hesitation; it's wise stewardship. It's choosing understanding over fear, and wisdom over impulse.

Throughout the years that I've coached others dealing with cancer, most did not initially take the time to educate. Not until the doctor said, "There's nothing more we can offer you."

When they hear those words, in desperation, they find me and learn what they could have learned at the very beginning of their journey. Fortunately, through good decisions and actions—even in their late stage, many win over cancer and recover their health.

Looking back, I see how my friend's advice reflects a spiritual principle: when we slow down, seek truth, and invite God into our decisions... clarity follows. Peace returns.

We Don't Know What We Don't Know

There's a common challenge in situations like cancer: people often don't realize what they don't know. They may feel confident that their understanding is accurate when, in reality, it's built on incomplete or incorrect information.

Unfortunately, when someone believes they already have the answers, they can become resistant to learning something new. This often happens after repeated exposure to false ideas that *feel* true.

It became imperative to ask the question: *What if there are things I haven't yet learned that could genuinely help me?*

What If "What I Know" Isn't True?

Shortly after being diagnosed with advanced-stage breast cancer, I no longer assumed that I had all the information needed. Learning to question what I thought I knew helped me more than words can say. The search for truth that began after a cancer diagnosis has continued until the current day. Learning to question and not stop until I find an unchanging, rock-solid truth saved my life—more than once.

In retrospect, one of the *best* decisions I ever made was to pause everything and educate myself.

Like most people, a lifetime of assumptions had been carried into that moment of diagnosis, beliefs shaped by culture, other people's stories and options, advertising, and fear-filled headlines.

Pause and Educate Yourself

Much of what felt like knowledge wasn't knowledge at

all. It was unexamined information—ideas absorbed over time without being questioned.

Sadly, misinformation had taken root over the decades and shaped my beliefs. Looking back, most of what I thought about cancer and chronic disease was wrong.

Scripture reminds us: *"My people are destroyed for lack of knowledge."* —Hosea 4:6

My husband, Dale, and I began spending time at the library. We both dug into medical journals and scientific papers. The focus shifted from collecting random information to asking real questions. The kind that leads to *real* answers.

What is cancer, really?

How does it develop and behave in the body?

Why did it show up in my life?

What caused it?

Most importantly, how can cancer be eliminated?

I also asked questions about standard cancer treatments.

What is chemotherapy, and what does it do to my body?

If the doctor removes my lymph nodes, what are the benefits and what are the negative side effects?

These questions became my starting point. Instead of surrendering to fear, my focus shifted to gaining knowledge and understanding, with the primary goal of pursuing what was true.

Scripture promises us, *"You shall know the truth, and the truth shall make you free."* —John 8:32

I am not ashamed of my belief that the Bible is God's Word and that Jesus is my Savior and Lord. Yet, this is not a book about the Bible. It's not about religion or the teachings of Jesus.

At the same time, it would be impossible for me to share my story without including some key Scriptures and principles that guided me.

The Bible tells us, *"I will praise You, for I am fearfully and wonderfully made."* —Psalm 139:14

I learned that my body was created to heal itself when it's cared for according to God's design.

The search for truth was slow at first. But finding answers allowed me to move forward with confidence.

You Have Time

After I was diagnosed, there was intense pressure to *do something*—and to do it quickly. It's likely you sense that too. Family, friends, doctors, and my emotions pushed for fast decisions and action.

After my own experience, and more than twenty years of helping others, I've learned that taking action matters. Usually, sooner is better than later.

But I've also learned that the most important first step is education and understanding—not rushing into drastic medical action.

Facts vs. Truth

Fortunately, before my diagnosis, I had learned that truth and facts are almost always different. Facts are based on observation and subjective interpretation of evidence that may or may not prove to be accurate. Truth is real and reliable—it's what faithfully reflects what is unchangeable. Because truth *never* changes.

Facts can change. But truth never changes.

And while I did not yet understand the full significance of what I was learning, something important was happening. Those early small discoveries began changing my incorrect beliefs about cancer. Old assumptions were starting to loosen, and for the first time, I was beginning to ask better questions.

What happened next would stretch my faith, challenge my thinking, and begin changing my path forward in unexpected ways. Looking back now, I can see that God was leading me step by step into discoveries that would alter the course of my life.

Chapter 4

What Cancer Is - What Cancer Is Not

A Quick Trip Back to the Beginning

"It's cancer," my doctor said in a matter-of-fact tone. "And it's aggressive. It's already spread too far. We couldn't get everything. You'll need another surgery—immediately."

He continued... laying out options, timelines, and next steps. Then came his warning: unless I strictly followed his recommended cancer protocol, aggressive chemo, radiation, and more surgery, my survival beyond three to six months would be almost impossible.

I quickly did the math. It was July.

Was he telling me I would likely not live to see Christmas?

I went into shock.

How was that possible? My body felt no weakness or sickness. On the outside, I still looked healthy. I felt pretty good. So how could something so deadly be inside me? How could my life so abruptly be in imminent danger?

Health had always seemed so easy... secure. At least, that was what I had always thought.

Suddenly, in an instant, everything seemed out of my control. Nothing was logical any longer.

I had always felt strong. Grounded. Capable. Confident in my future.

Now it felt like I was standing on a slippery slope, struggling to keep my balance.

What was solid? Nothing about my life seemed familiar anymore. I looked at the doctor, the room around me, and was terrified.

My focus narrowed to one simple thought:

Get the cancer out of my body!

Cut it out.

Remove it.

Fix the problem.

That's all I wanted.

That's all I understood at the time.

I was definitely in reaction mode.

We scheduled my next surgery for the first available date.

The doctor was highly experienced, well respected, and deeply knowledgeable in cancer treatment. Just as important, he was warm, kind, and approachable. Based upon my understanding at the time, I felt safe in his care.

During the days of waiting for surgery, I gained valuable insight through new friendships. I sought out others further along in their cancer journeys. Some had lived with cancer for months, others for years. Listening to their stories answered questions I didn't yet know to ask.

Some were in active treatment. Others were in remission. I asked each one what they were thankful they had done—and what, in hindsight, they wished they had done differently. This helped me gain tremendous insight into the choices I was facing.

Hearing their stories made me realize that every choice mattered, and that clarity didn't come easily—or quickly.

Time was running away from me. Just when I needed it to slow down, my days were rushing forward, leaving barely any room to process what was happening.

There were appointments with my oncologist. Wig shopping with my husband, emotional preparation for a future that included more surgery, chemotherapy, and radiation.

A Setback That Felt Like Defeat

When the next surgery arrived, I felt confident that all the cancer would finally be removed. At that point, I still believed eliminating the tumor would cure the cancer and restore my health.

Going back under the knife came with the expectation of waking up to good news. But that's not at all what happened.

Instead, after the surgery, consciousness returned with the doctor gently slapping my cheek, forcing me out of the drug-induced haze of anesthesia. His face came into focus, reflecting a worry I didn't expect or understand. And what he said, I wasn't prepared to hear.

"Paula, we had to abort. We couldn't do the surgery," he said matter-of-factly.

"We found a severe staph infection, no doubt caused by the first biopsy. We had to close you back up. We'll place you on strong antibiotics for thirty days, and then we can try again."

My heart sank.

Are you kidding me? Did I hear that correctly?

Is he saying that cancer is still growing inside of me?

Still growing.

Still spreading.
Still threatening my life.

I poured out my questions to God—along with my fear and even my anger. This didn't feel like progress at all. It felt like I was losing ground, as if everything I had fought so hard for was slipping away.

What I couldn't see at that moment was that the next thirty days *of waiting* would become one of the most important seasons of my life.

Let me share something deeply personal. My desire is always to be honest—to tell the truth, even when it reveals my own weaknesses.

Although a trusted friend, doctor, and cancer specialist previously encouraged me to pause and fully understand my options, I still rushed ahead with the already scheduled surgery.

My belief that the cancer had to be removed from my body as quickly as possible felt urgent and unquestionable. Added to that was the constant pressure from my doctor and from many of those who loved me—to take immediate action.

In what I can only describe as God's mercy, that second surgery was blocked. Looking back, I see how patiently the Lord Jesus guided me, even when I wasn't fully listening.

"Trust in the Lord with all your heart, and lean not on your own understanding; In all your ways acknowledge Him, And He shall direct your paths." —Proverbs 3:5

God was teaching me something important. I needed to trust His timing and His direction—not my own sense of urgency or others' opinions. I share this humbly, not as someone who had it all figured out, but simply as part of my journey.

If there is anything I learned along the way, even in my missteps, that can help you, it brings me both gratitude and joy.

Of course, it's always better to go God's way from the beginning. But God is gracious, and He can redeem even our hurried or foolish choices.

In my desperation, I brought my diagnosis to the Lord and committed to follow His leading one step at a time. I realized I was not facing the battle alone. Heaven's help was real, and God was present with me.

The Delay That Became Direction

What began as a panic-driven delay of the surgery soon became something entirely different. The pause in my treatment gave me desperately needed time to search for answers to the questions right in front of me.

God had not made a mistake.

He was answering my prayers.

During those thirty pivotal days of delay, my

husband and I were at the library nearly every day. We studied medical journals, research papers, reports, and statistics—anything related to cancer and the aggressive treatments my doctor proposed.

A few days later, shocking information surfaced. I knew it was the truth. What was discovered changed everything I had always believed about cancer.

My tumor was not the cancer!

I was dumbfounded.

The malignant tumor was only a *symptom* of cancer. Something much deeper was happening inside my body. I was learning that the tumor was only a physical indication of a systemic condition.

The tumor is not the cancer.

With that new understanding, I realized that if the doctor removed the entire tumor, it wouldn't fix my problem. Cancer would still be developing in my body. For me, this revelation changed everything.

One day earlier, before this discovery, I believed that if the tumor were removed, the cancer would be out of my body. But armed with new information, I realized the cause of my tumor would still be present to create more tumors.

Still reeling from the new awareness that cancer is not the tumor, a bigger question arose.

So, if the tumor isn't the cancer, what is?

I kept searching to better understand. My heart raced as I flipped through one journal after another and read everything that might lead me to the answer I needed. Finally, I found what I was searching for. The information shocked me. Could it be true?

Cancer is my own damaged cells.

What? Cancer is my own cells that have somehow been damaged? How had I not known this?

Finally, for the first time, I understood what cancer really is... and what it is not.

I had always believed cancer was a foreign invader. Now I was learning that cancer started within my own body when my cells had been damaged.

Why had no one ever explained this?

These discoveries were doing more than reshaping my beliefs about cancer. I was sensing the possibility of regaining control over my own life again.

Cancer doesn't come from an outside invader.
Cancer is our own damaged cells.

With each new revelation, my understanding expanded. My perspective of what was true began to adjust. But every answer seemed to open the door to another unsettling question.

What had gone wrong inside my body that caused my own cells to turn against me...

and become deadly?

It became very important for me to understand *why* I got cancer. That question of why became my new focus. Because until I addressed the root causes, nothing would really change.

As I dug deeper, it became clear that a battle was taking place inside my body—a battle between healthy cells and damaged cells. With greater knowledge came greater clarity and growing confidence that the disease could be overcome.

Signs of Danger Before the Storm

As I looked at my past, it became clear that without realizing it, I had been undermining my health for years—not deliberately, but unknowingly.

In simple terms, my fast-paced lifestyle had left me living on empty calories, too much caffeine that kept my body chronically dehydrated, and constant stress that I had ignored for far too long.

The negative factors were surprisingly simple and painfully familiar.

Chronic dehydration—not enough pure water and far too much caffeine, leaving my body constantly depleted of hydration.

Poor nutrition—depriving my body of the nutrients it truly needed. I was unintentionally denying my cells the building blocks they need for health, strength, and healing, and asking my body to perform without properly fueling it.

Unmanaged stress—relentlessly flooding my body with harmful stress hormones that steadily wore down my defenses.

None of this happened overnight. It was the slow accumulation of everyday habits. But together, they weakened my immune system and created the perfect environment for illness to take hold.

These were only the most obvious contributors that helped lay the groundwork for the disease. The more I learned about what damages cells and weakens the immune system, the more my cancer diagnosis made sense.

My body had not suddenly betrayed me. It had been sending warning signals for a long time—signals I hadn't learned to recognize.

CHAPTER 5

The Root Problem

Learning about the body and how it heals reveals a simple truth: the human body is constantly working to restore health and stay alive.

Beneath the surface, trillions of tiny cells repair damage, replace worn tissue, and defend against threats. Entire systems rebuild themselves day after day. Much of this work happens without effort or even awareness. This healing design was built into the body from the beginning.

Healthy Cells vs. Damaged Cells

I learned that the human body contains roughly thirty to forty trillion cells—an astonishing number. Each one was created to play a role in maintaining life. Many are red blood cells that carry oxygen throughout the body.

Others form skin, muscle, nerves, and the immune system. Together, they work continuously to repair, renew, and protect the body.

None of it remains still. This vast network is always moving. Cells die, and new ones take their place. Moment by moment, the body rebuilds itself through a built-in, God-created operating system.

Each healthy cell arrives with a purpose. A pre-programmed assignment. A natural lifespan. It does its work, replaces itself, then quietly exits, making room for what comes next.

But a cell that's been damaged performs differently. It's important to understand because these damaged cells are what make up cancer.

I discovered that in a damaged cell, the DNA instructions have been negatively altered. When that happens, the cell no longer follows its original design. It stops contributing. It no longer serves any useful purpose. It continues to multiply. And as it divides, it creates more of its kind, with the same faulty DNA instructions.

Healthy cells have built-in instructions that control how long they live and when they should die.

But cancer cells can lose that directive. Without a signal to stop growing or die off, they continue multiplying uncontrollably, keep dividing, build upon one another, and, over time, form a tumor.

A damaged cell's DNA instruction changes, causing it to stop helping, no longer die, and continue to multiply until it forms a tumor.

These damaged cells take up space. They drain resources. They steal nutrients and energy meant for healthy cells, while placing added strain on the already weak immune system.

The immune system must work harder to recognize, repair, and destroy these abnormal cells. But when damaged cells continue multiplying unchecked, the body's burden increases. Pressure builds over time, and if the immune system is already weak, it can eventually become overwhelmed.

That's when it finally hit me. Cancer wasn't some foreign thing invading my body. It was a group of my own injured cells—cells that malfunctioned, refused to die, and continued multiplying. When enough of them gather together, it is called 'cancer'.

What I just described is *what cancer is.*

This deeper understanding made me aware that I was standing on the edge of something powerful. I was finally understanding how my body was designed to function, and what happens when cells become damaged.

First came the shock that a tumor isn't cancer—it's a symptom.

Then came the realization that cancer is not a

foreign invader. Cancer is made of my own damaged cells.

And finally, another piece of the cancer puzzle surfaced: Cancer is a systemic disease.

Cancer is Systemic: What Does That Mean?

I wanted to understand why this was so important, so I kept digging. The reason cancer is called *systemic* is that it doesn't just affect the spot where it starts. Cancer involves the entire body—organs, systems, energy, and the immune system. Everything.

Cancer is a systemic disease.

Even when a tumor begins in one area, such as the breast, lung, or colon, cancer cells can break away and travel through the bloodstream or lymph system to take root in other parts of the body. That process, called metastasis, made the disease feel far more serious and complex to me.

Then I discovered another surprise—one that required an additional shift in my thinking.

The Solution to the problem

Everyone develops damaged cells from time to time. Everyone. It's a normal occurrence inside the body. The difference lies in the immune system's health—whether it is strong enough to recognize and remove damaged cells before they multiply and cause harm.

I realized I could not simply remove a tumor and expect everything to return to normal.

As I thought about a tumor in light of my new understanding, it reminded me of a weed in a garden. You can cut the weed off at the surface, but if the root remains, the weed grows back. Removing what is visible does not solve the deeper problem beneath the surface.

Cancer works the same way. Shrinking or removing tumors alone doesn't correct the conditions that allowed them to grow in the first place.

Removing a tumor doesn't correct the problem that allowed it to grow in the first place.

The real issue was deeper than a tumor, which is only a symptom of the problem.

It was time to become proactive instead of defensive.

Research and medical journals filled my days. But gradually, clarity replaced the hopelessness of feeling overwhelmed. Cancer became more understandable. Less mysterious.

The deeper I dug, the more it felt like peeling back the layers of an onion. Each new layer revealed something I hadn't understood before.

From Fear to Informed Decisions

By the end of thirty days of non-stop study, self-education, and research, something remarkable had happened.

I was no longer operating from panic or reacting out of fear.

I was able to make informed decisions based on reality. And making choices based on truth would ultimately alter my course and save my life.

The truths I was discovering made sense. My confidence and sense of control were returning.

If cancer had developed through misuse and neglect, it seemed logical that reversing those patterns could reverse the cancer in my body.

For the first time, I understood that my health was not simply a matter of chance. I had to take responsibility for what was happening in my body, including the cancer itself.

Medicine had a role—to support what I couldn't do on my own. In the end, its role would be minimal.

God designed my body with the ability to heal itself, yet I had unknowingly worked against His design.

My depleted immune system needed rebuilding. Fast. This new understanding created a turning point in my journey.

Chapter 6

Created to Heal

At this point in my journey, I became convinced that cancer had taken hold in my body when my depleted immune system was no longer functioning in the way it was designed.

If my immune system could be strengthened again, and quickly, perhaps my body could heal naturally.

I learned that the immune system is designed to function like an internal security force that constantly scans for damaged cells and other internal threats, repairing what can be restored and removing what doesn't belong. Quietly and faithfully, it works day and night to protect the body.

But in my case, it seemed that through years of neglect and strain, that system had slowly weakened. Little by little, the very defense system created to protect me had nearly stopped functioning, allowing disease to settle in and grow in my body.

About two years earlier, I had gone through an intensely stressful season. I came to believe it was the tipping point of profoundly weakening my immune system.

During my research, I learned that cancer is often not detected until years after a tumor begins to grow. That timeline gave new weight to the stress I had experienced, casting that earlier trauma in a more ominous light.

It also deepened my understanding of how powerfully chronic stress can work against the body's health.

My top priority had become strengthening my immune system. Improving my body's natural defenses moved to the front of everything I was doing.

Eye-Opening Discoveries

Along the way, a deeper study of cancer and of how the human body functions revealed one truth after another. And each discovery encouraged me forward in my quest for healing.

Discovering how dramatically cancer rates in the United States have risen over the past century was eye-opening.

Our environment has dramatically changed. Our

food has altered. Our daily habits have adapted to modern living—but not in good ways that support our health.

The human body was never designed to handle many of these shifts within our modern culture. As those changes increased, vulnerability to disease grew alongside them.

Much of what we eat today is highly processed and man-made. You've likely heard the phrase "empty calories," referring to foods that provide energy but very little true nourishment. Over time, I realized that many modern foods have been stripped of vital nutrients. So that even when feeling full, my body wasn't truly receiving what it needed to thrive.

Learning what the body actually requires for health was suddenly on my radar.

Fresh vegetables, fruits, and whole foods—simple foods that are unprocessed and free from additives began to make a noticeable difference. My energy improved. My body felt more balanced. A sense of well-being slowly returned.

It became clear that the foods God placed on this earth were not just meant to fill our stomachs—they were designed to nourish the bodies He created—much like putting the right fuel into a car's gas tank. Returning to those natural foods gave my body a foundation for healing that I had not experienced before.

My new approach to natural health was to bring my body back into alignment with God's design. And this was allowing my body to restore and heal.

Fear Left - Hope Returned

Before my diagnosis, cancer had always been a mystery to both my husband and me. Like many families, we had watched dozens of loved ones suffer from the disease. Yet we never really tried to understand it. The hope was simply that we would never become one of the "unlucky ones."

But as I continued learning more about cancer and my body, something surprising happened. Instead of feeling overwhelmed, motivation began to grow.

It was becoming clear that cancer reflected cause-and-effect. Fear slowly began to lose its grip, and helplessness gave way to hope as clear, practical steps emerged for rebuilding the immune system and restoring health.

A future filled with healthy living and meaningful purpose came back into view.

The body is remarkably resilient. Yet because healing naturally is a gradual process, it requires time, support, and proper care. In my case, symptoms became worse before they began to improve. This makes sense to me now, but back then... it was a challenge to trust and continue my course.

Healing certainly did not happen overnight. It unfolded slowly and deliberately. I began to understand that after years of decline, reversing that course took time.

At least, that is how my healing unfolded... slowly, gradually. Over time, my immune system strengthened enough to begin doing its job once again—attacking the cancerous cells in my body.

As I continued to intentionally rebuild my immune system, little by little, the tide shifted. And what once threatened my life began to steadily retreat—until eighteen months later, the cancer was completely gone.

That was more than twenty-five years ago.

Since then, life has been free from both cancer and the fear that once surrounded it—not because the illness was ignored, but because the *truth* was discovered. That truth brought understanding, enabling wiser choices and leading to a better, permanent outcome.

Today, I have the privilege of walking alongside others who have received a cancer diagnosis. It is an honor to support them as they begin their own journey toward healing—body, soul, and spirit.

And if you have recently received a diagnosis, you may be feeling what I once felt: confusion, fear, and an urgent need for answers.

Please know you are not alone.

There is a path forward, even when the road ahead

seems uncertain. With patience, wisdom, and faith, restoration can begin. Permanent lasting health can be yours.

Obviously, I chose the path less traveled—to heal my body naturally. That choice also meant that I would not proceed with the medical system's recommended protocol—more surgery, chemo, and radiation.

My doctor's statement, that I would likely be dead in three to six months if I didn't aggressively pursue the treatments he recommended, became less powerful as new facts were discovered, and my understanding was renewed.

There is still so much more to share. And truly, the best is yet to come.

Chapter 7

Healing Your Body, Soul & Spirit

For most of my life, I had thought of health in only one way—the physical body. If something was wrong, the body must be the problem. But during my journey through cancer, an unexpected discovery began to change that thinking.

The human being is far more complex than flesh and bone. In addition to the physical body are two other parts of our being that influence health every day. Once this became clear, many aspects of healing began to make more sense.

This chapter is close to my heart. Gaining an understanding of the body, soul, and spirit changed my life as much as anything in this book. Every single day, I benefit from the revelation that I am a spirit. I have a soul. And I live in a body.

Sickness and Health Are Not Only Physical

After discovering more about what cancer is and how it behaves within the body, my perspective on how to regain my health was transformed. Then my attention turned more inward, as it became increasingly clear that the soul and spirit also played a vital role in my healing journey.

Over time, I could see a pattern. Many illnesses—especially cancer—can often be traced back to deeper wounds carried inside. Wounds that reside in what Scripture calls the soul.

It isn't that a past trauma directly causes cancer. Rather, unresolved trauma or stress gradually weakens the immune system, creating a vulnerability in the body where disease can take hold.

In my case, it eventually became clear that a major stress I experienced a couple of years earlier had become, as the saying goes, the straw that broke the camel's back.

My immune system had already been weakened for many of the reasons I previously shared. But when this major stress occurred over a period of several months, it caused toxic stress hormones to be released into my body 24/7. This acute stress of my already compromised immune system proved to be more than my body could handle.

It's also important to understand that the moment of diagnosis is not when cancer actually begins. A diagnosis means the disease has progressed to the point where it can be detected.

In my case, the tumor had likely been growing for a couple of years before it became large enough to 'feel,' thus prompting a doctor's visit, which led to my diagnosis.

Injury to the Soul

The Bible teaches that the soul contains a person's mind, will, and emotions. Damage to the soul due to unresolved trauma or stress often contributes to cancer or other diseases through increased weakening of the immune system.

The soul is the place where thoughts live, where choices are made, and where feelings are processed. It is also where pain and abuse can settle. It is where trauma wounds remain, and where unforgiveness stubbornly puts down roots.

Stress, trauma, hurt, and unforgiveness all begin in the soul—but they don't stay there. They spill over into the physical, weakening the immune system and disrupting the body's ability to heal.

The Discovery that Helped Me Heal

Years earlier, my husband, Dale, was the sole survivor of a horrific airplane crash. Seconds after impact, something extraordinary happened.

Hovering several feet above the crash site, he saw his own body lying below—lifeless. In that moment, he realized he was not his body. He was a spirit—still alive —more than ever.

He suddenly understood something that would change everything: he is a spirit, he has a soul, and he once lived in that body below.

In that instant, he also knew that every person is created by God in three parts: spirit, soul, and body.

That experience stayed with him. I learned from it. And during my cancer journey, its meaning became abundantly clear.

Complete and permanent healing isn't one-dimensional.

(Dale's experience and what he learned are shared in his books: *Atomic Faith* and *Visiting Heaven*.)

Dale shared this revelation with me years earlier, but during my battle with cancer, it took on a deeper, more powerful meaning. Understanding my three-part being—body, soul, and spirit—gave me a foundation that could not easily be shaken. I realized there were tools within my soul and spirit to help me win the battle in my physical body.

The Whole Person: Body, Soul, and Spirit

People are much more than just physical bodies. The soul and spirit affect how a person lives, thinks, and experiences life.

My **body** is the outer, visible layer. It interacts with the physical world through my senses—seeing, hearing, tasting, touching, and smelling. It is a temporary vehicle for the soul and spirit, like a car that takes me through life. Other people see my physical body and recognize me, but I am much more than my body.

My **soul** is the interface between my body and spirit. It is where thoughts are formed, information is processed, choices are made, and feelings are experienced. The soul shapes attitudes, beliefs, and responses to life. It determines what words I speak and what actions I take.

The soul is eternal and will never cease to exist, but will take the lessons learned during my earthly journey into eternity.

My **spirit** is the real me. In fact, I was created as a spirit—first and foremost. It is through my spirit that I can connect with God and receive eternal life. According to the Bible, I will never die but will live forever.

Every person is created as an eternal spirit.
Each person has an eternal soul.
All people live temporarily in a physical body.

These three parts—spirit, soul, and body—are closely interconnected. What happens in one part influences the others. When these three parts work together in harmony, the foundation for health becomes much stronger.

We are all spiritual beings
having a human experience.

For me, what once seemed deeply insightful became lifesaving. When I began to apply this understanding to my own healing journey, everything shifted.

It changed how I fought my battle.

It changed how I cared for myself.

It changed how I engaged with faith for healing from God.

The body–soul–spirit perspective is not a new revelation. It's woven throughout Scripture from beginning to end. Once this insight became clear, it was impossible for me to overlook.

In Genesis 1:26, we learn: *"Then God said, "Let Us make man in Our image, according to Our likeness;"* I believe God created mankind in His image—spirit, soul, and body—each part divinely designed and interconnected.

Physical healing unfolds more freely when body, soul, and spirit are brought into harmony with God's original design.

Gradually, it became clear... it wasn't just my body that needed healing.

It was *all* of me.

"Now may the God of peace Himself sanctify you completely; and may your whole spirit, soul, and body be preserved blameless at the coming of our Lord Jesus Christ."

—1 Thessalonians 5:23

All of Me Needed Healing

There is much more to explore about the powerful relationship between the body, soul, and spirit. And I address these in greater detail in the *Winning Over Cancer Coaching Program*. Yet, because this subject is so vital, let's look at some basics here.

The Body and My Healing Journey

When the cancer diagnosis arrived, life was full. Busy. Active. Moving at a steady pace. Like so many others, my focus stayed on what could be seen—my body. Yet, little attention was given to what was happening deep inside.

Minor illnesses had always been handled with over-the-counter remedies. Or, when needed... a doctor's visit.

My husband and I were entrepreneurs, building several companies together. Little time was spent considering how personal stewardship of my body affected my overall health.

Life moved forward under the assumption that my body would take care of itself.

What wasn't understood at the time was how deeply the choices I made every day were shaping my health. Chronic dehydration. Poor food choices. Stress. Rest—or the lack of it. And the way I handled my emotions. All of it silently influences my future.

My body isn't just something I live in. It's something I've been entrusted with. A gift. A treasure that deserves care, attention, and stewardship.

Today, we live in a culture obsessed with health, yet we are somehow sicker and heavier than ever. Information is everywhere. Supplements line the shelves. Yet still, chronic illnesses keep rising. And so do cancer rates.

As I learned how my body works, things began to make more sense. Previously, I had little awareness of what my body needed to remain strong and healthy. And without that knowledge, I became vulnerable.

In today's modern, toxic environment, chronic disease has become increasingly common. For many people, it is no longer a question of *whether* illness will come, but *when*.

The Spirit and My Healing Journey

Fortunately, even before cancer was discovered in my body, I had already formed a connection with God through my relationship with Jesus Christ.

Since God created and designed my body, it seemed clear that He could also help me restore it to permanent health.

Through poor stewardship, I had allowed myself to drift out of alignment with His design. It was my responsibility to bring it back.

How God Heals

Like many Christians, when I was first diagnosed, I prayed for healing. That was my immediate response. I knew God was able. But if I'm honest, I didn't fully understand how He heals or how to receive that healing.

Along the way, that began to change.

Little by little, I started to see that healing wasn't as complicated as I had once thought. But it also wasn't as casual as simply hoping it would happen. There was a deeper understanding that God began to reveal to me. And as that understanding grew, so did my confidence.

I came to realize that healing is not reserved for a select few. It isn't something God gives to some and withholds from others. What Jesus provided through His finished work is far more powerful than I had previously understood. Healing had already been made available.

What needed to change... was me.

Not in a way of striving or earning—but in learning how to come into agreement with God. He is constant. He does not change. But I had to learn to align my thinking, my beliefs, and my responses with His truth.

Three key things became very clear to me.

I needed to become fully convinced that it is God's will to heal. And that He does not play favorites. Only then could my "belief" become rooted enough to produce faith.

It was also necessary that I understand *how to receive from God.*

Before this, I had approached healing in ways that felt incomplete. At times, I hoped God would heal me. Other times, I thought maybe if I could believe strongly enough, it would happen. And deep down, there were even moments when I wondered if I needed to somehow deserve it.

But through this journey, I began to see something different.

Healing does not come from striving, earning, or hoping. But from understanding what God has already provided, and learning how to receive.

Scripture has much to say about the strength and stability that come when the body, soul, and spirit are brought into harmony with God's design.

As I began thinking about my body, healing, and my responsibility to live the way God intended, I realized everything was connected. That true healing was not just physical.

The Soul and My Healing Journey

Every choice, action, and word begins in the soul. My mind, will, and emotions shape how I think, feel, and respond to life. Very quickly, I realized that understanding and learning to manage this part of myself would greatly influence my outcome over cancer. And it did.

Without renewing my mind, my soul naturally drifted toward the patterns and thinking of the world around me. It was easy to accept what culture considered normal. But God created the whole person to function best when the soul is aligned with the spirit, and the spirit is aligned with Him.

An additional Scripture brought this truth home for me:

"For as a man thinks in his heart, so is he..." — Proverbs 23:7

The power of thought is real and can be life-changing. Since every part of the soul begins with thought, I gradually began to recognize how important my thinking patterns were. Little by little, my thoughts started to change. Old ways of thinking gave way to new ones.

Thoughts affected my emotions, my decisions, and ultimately the direction of my life. Instead of working against healing, my new thought patterns began to support it.

But keep in mind, the soul also carries hidden burdens.

Emotional wounds.

Past trauma.

Unresolved hurts.

Unhealed wounds remained buried deep inside. Quietly draining peace. Stealing joy and placing invisible strain on my body. They were also shaping my beliefs, while quietly limiting what I felt was possible.

Along the way, I began to gain deeper clarity about the causes of my cancer.

There were deep wounds to acknowledge and resolve.

Issues to confront.

People to forgive.

The more I learned, the more amazed I became at

how closely the three parts of my being are connected. Spirit, soul, and body are constantly influencing one another—for good or for harm.

Three-Part Harmony

The soul is the bridge between the spirit and the body. It connects the eternal with the temporary physical—the spiritual with the natural.

When these three parts work together, as they were designed to, the result is powerful whole-person harmony. And the results compound.

Although the body is temporary, it is precious. God had entrusted me with a body to nurture, protect, and honor. The choices made in caring for it influence how long my life on earth may be.

Scripture reminded me:

"For You formed my inward parts; ... I will praise You, for I am fearfully and wonderfully made; Marvelous are Your works, And that my soul knows very well."
—Psalm 139:13–14

Because God created each part of me—body, soul, and spirit—learning to care for my whole person His way became essential.

As my body, soul, and spirit came back into harmony with God's design, healing began to flow naturally and rapidly.

**By bringing the body, soul, and spirit
into harmony with God's design,
healing follows naturally.**

But this was not the end of the story. It was the point at which regaining health truly began to gain momentum.

Chapter 8

Choosing To Live

During my battle with cancer, fear was often an unwelcome companion that refused to leave. It was a bully that continued to assault my peace, and my belief that the battle with cancer could be won. Fear showed up in quiet moments, whispering questions I didn't want to face: *What if my approach fails? What if things get worse? What if I don't make it?*

Many mornings, I woke up already tired from the battle in my mind. Yet beneath all that noise, something stronger was growing in my heart. God's Word reminded me that life is not meant to be surrendered to fear or chance. Repeatedly, I heard the same gentle instruction: *Choose life.* Slowly, I realized—this was a decision that only I could make.

Yet, it surprised me how—for a reason I couldn't understand—it felt like, under the circumstances, I didn't have the right or the power to make that choice. Somewhere in the space between fear and faith, a decision had to be made. I knew how important *choosing* was in any battle of faith. Life doesn't happen by accident. It is chosen. Chosen on purpose—one thought, one word, one brave step at a time.

I finally realized that I couldn't avoid this decision or delay it. *Not* deciding was a decision *not* to choose life.

Choosing is a powerful thing, a spiritual force. I could use it to my advantage or let it work against me.

Scripture tells us something important:

"I call heaven and earth as witnesses today against you, that I have set before you life and death, blessing and cursing; therefore choose life, that both you and your descendants may live." —Deuteronomy 30:19

When circumstances feel overwhelming, something sacred and powerful still remains within reach for every one of us: the ability to choose life. But choosing life is not a one-time decision. It is a choice we must make repeatedly, every single day.

Choice requires action to release faith, because faith is the force that helps bring a choice into fulfillment.

Faith is the force that helps bring a choice into fulfillment.

Once I decided to choose life, I realized I also

needed to act like I truly believed life and healing were possible.

Truth Outweighs Facts

When cancer entered my world, I quickly learned there was a difference between facts, statistics, and truth. They are not the same. Facts and stats can change. Prognosis can shift. But the truth is what is real. Truth remains constant. It never changes.

My doctor explained what the tests revealed. Those were facts. He backed them up with statistics, as he told me what was needed.

But as I listened to numbers describe my future, something happened. I knew in my heart I was not hearing the truth. I had known for decades that God leads His people to the truth. I'd witnessed God do this for me dozens of times before.

Medical stats are important. Cancer protocols are real. But for me, I knew God was already opening my eyes to see things differently—the way He saw them.

God had consistently been leading me toward truth—beyond the endless facts and reports coming from every direction. And there was confidence He would continue, because His wisdom was being sought diligently, and truth was more important to me than fear-filled facts.

As prayer for truth continued, faith consistently responded with action based on what was believed. Both experience and Scripture became evidence that God answers prayer where genuine faith exists.

So, I expected something more powerful than the medical data I was seeing and hearing would be revealed. Truth is real. And truth does not change. It was true then. And it remains true now.

A life-threatening diagnosis has a way of stripping away everything familiar. Yet there was confidence that God had a way through. He always does. I believe God wants to lead His people to victory... always. But knowing that required a willingness to follow the path He set before me. That part was not always easy.

I knew that truth wasn't found in test results or prognosis. It was found in God's Word. So, I leaned hard on Scripture, about God's faithfulness, about His desire to heal. About my choice to live.

God's Word reminded me over and over of what He had already provided:

"...who Himself bore our sins in His own body on the tree, that we, having died to sins, might live for righteousness—by whose stripes you were healed."
—1 Peter 2:24 (author emphasis)

"Who forgives all your iniquities,
Who heals all your diseases,
Who redeems your life from destruction,

Who crowns you with lovingkindness and tender mercies;" —Psalms 103:3–4 (author emphasis)

God's promises stood alongside the medical facts—and the choice was mine to make. What would I believe? Who would I trust? This was my turning point.

In my heart, I made a final decision.

I chose to trust God.

I chose to believe His Word.

I chose to live.

This wasn't positive thinking or religious language. It was a deliberate choice to place God's Word as the final authority in my battle with cancer.

When Facts and Truth Collide

It was unavoidable... the collision. Two sides warring from opposite perspectives. With contradicting evidence. And I was caught in the middle.

The numbers surrounding cancer can feel overwhelming. Every day, more than 5,000 people receive a diagnosis, and on average,1,700 lives are lost. Those realities are sobering. And they're real.

But a diagnosis need not define the outcome. In light of God's promises, becoming a statistic was not an option for me.

What *did* matter was understanding what I was facing and choosing not to surrender my future to the stats and reports.

This wasn't about will-power alone, but by choosing what I believed was true and then acting on that belief with faith. I had to pick a side.

Statistically speaking, I learned that one out of every two men and one out of every three women will develop cancer in their lifetime. With figures like these, it became even more important to learn what was true for myself, rather than relying solely on what others say or predict. After all, it was my life.

Statistics report that one out of every two men and one out of every three women will develop cancer in their lifetime.

The realization of what I faced became clear—every day, I had to choose life. Not simply because I wanted to live, but because I knew God was asking me to choose Him. And where God is, there is life.

That decision led to a deeper question: what path leads to life?

Scripture gave me that answer: *"Death and life are in the power of the tongue..."*

—Proverbs 18:21

God gives promises, but those promises require a response—agreement in both word and action.

Faith is not passive. Faith is acting on what you believe.

A major part of my ultimate success began with the

decision to choose life. Once my choice was made, my thoughts, words, and actions turned toward living—focused on health and healing.

Faith is not passive.
Faith is acting on what you believe.

At first, it felt like herding cats. But with continued commitment, gradually bringing my thoughts, words, and actions into alignment became easier until a steady daily pattern emerged.

Speaking as though a wonderful future lay ahead. Planning as though that future was secure. Acting in agreement with those declarations. This was forward motion. This was faith in action, rooted in truth.

God's promises filled my mind. Health was spoken with every word. Thoughts, words, and actions gradually came into agreement with the choice to live and with God's design for the body.

Restored health was chosen and believed in my heart—every day, even every hour. It became reality. Believed, spoken, and acted upon as though it were already true.

Emotions had to take a back seat. They shouted warnings. Tried to convince me the path was wrong. Again, and again—thoughts and feelings attempted to open the door to fear.

But every day, the choice to live was made... and I just kept choosing.

Chapter 9

Restoring Health Daily

There came a moment in my self-education when I realized I had to do more than learn. It was time to put into action the truths I had found and assume personal responsibility toward actively rebuilding my health.

It started with not just identifying and removing what was harming my health but also rebuilding what had been weakened—specifically, my immune system.

Daily choices became actions, starting with what I ate and drank. It was time to take responsibility for everything that went into my body. My new identity as the manager of my health included monitoring: hydration, nutrition, movement, reducing toxin exposure, lifestyle habits, and managing stress. Every decision either moved my body closer to health or further away from it. These weren't abstract ideas anymore. They became part of my daily recovery process.

Nourishing the Body

By learning what nourishes the body, something unsettling became clear. Much of what was considered *normal* was far different from the foods God designed to feed us.

Convenience had replaced nourishment. Many foods were engineered to cause cravings or addiction rather than satisfaction. Most of the modern choices had nothing to do with restoring or maintaining health, even what was labeled healthy.

Another realization followed: it was possible to be well-fed and still undernourished. Calories and macronutrients were easy to find, yet vital nutrients needed for repair and healing were often missing from the foods I had lived on. A full plate did not always mean a nourished body.

It is possible to be well-fed and still undernourished.

In the past, when I chose something to eat, it was about whether I liked the taste or *wanted* it, rather than what it provided my body in terms of health.

When cells are deprived of what they need and

burdened with what they cannot use, the effects accumulate over time, weakening the immune system and undermining the body's ability to heal.

The Body is Created to Heal

Extra Weight

Modern diets often lead to excess weight, which places constant strain on the body and weakens immune health. In Western culture, a major contributor is the steady consumption of *empty calories.* These are foods that supply energy but little nourishment. I learned that eliminating processed foods and choosing natural, whole foods truly supported my health.

Lifestyle

The typical American lifestyle impacts our health just as much as diet does. Excessive alcohol, smoking, and long-term exposure to medications all weaken the immune system and place added stress on the body.

In addition, chronic dehydration is far more common than most people realize. I discovered it is often caused by consuming too much caffeine—or simply not drinking enough water.

I was under the impression that my hydration was adequate because of the large amount of coffee and soda consumed. However, liquid is not the same as water. Learning that every caffeinated beverage requires approximately two glasses of water to replace what the body uses to process a single cup of caffeinated coffee or soda was a wake-up call. With that information, it became immediately clear that I was in the category of "chronically dehydrated."

Healthy Cells Need Oxygen

Oxygen is a critical component in a healthy cell. Movement helps oxygen reach every part of the body. Deeper breathing during activity carries oxygen through the bloodstream to the cells. Circulation improves. Detoxification is supported. The immune system is strengthened. And the body's natural healing processes are awakened.

The body was never designed for long hours of inactivity. Earlier generations stayed active simply through the demands of daily life—walking, lifting, working, and moving. Today, far too much time is spent sitting in cars, behind desks, or in front of screens. It became clear that my lifestyle needed to change.

Every cell in the body requires adequate oxygen to remain healthy. Without it, the cell can become damaged. I was learning.

The dots began to connect—the principles I learned about damaged cells directly influenced the way the body is managed. My focus expanded not only to feeding my body but also to nourishing my cells.

Stress Becomes Impossible to Ignore

When people pursue better health, they often focus on diet, medicine, or environment. Yet one of the greatest health threats often goes unaddressed—stress. This "killer" silently weakens the immune system, opening the door to disease.

The role stress played in my life hadn't fully been understood until after my diagnosis. For years, my life had been in the fast lane as a business owner, wife, mother, and someone with a full social calendar. The constant pressure felt normal.

Through an honest evaluation of my lifestyle, I identified multiple sources that had depleted my health: work demands, relationships, financial concerns, and the constant weight of daily responsibilities.

Physical stressors were also present, including dehydration, malnutrition, exposure to environmental toxins, and inadequate rest.

Sometimes the problem runs even deeper: unresolved trauma, hurt, grief, or holding onto unforgiveness.

Along the way, I discovered that a major emotional

or physical trauma can become a tipping point. Such events often further drain an already weakened immune system, reducing the body's natural defenses to a point of vulnerability.

A major emotional or physical trauma can become a tipping point for disease.

When the body becomes weakened, abnormal cells may begin multiplying faster than the immune system can control them. Over time, this unchecked growth can lead to tumor formation.

Recognizing these patterns helped me make the changes needed to manage stress.

Cancer's Invisible Emotional Triggers

Past trauma, bitterness, or unforgiveness may seem like closed chapters. Yet when emotional wounds are not fully healed, they continue to affect the body in subtle but negative ways.

Because this type of stress operates beneath the surface, it can slowly weaken the immune system like a silent attacker. Even when the mind has moved on, the body remembers.

This realization revealed an important truth—the spirit, soul, and body are deeply interconnected. When one is wounded, the others are often affected and reflect the damage in some way.

Prolonged stress affects more than emotions. It ultimately impacts the body through the release of toxic stress hormones. This consistent bombardment weakens the immune system and drains health and strength.

Healing is still possible, but not without reducing and managing stress.

One of the most difficult decisions in my journey was stepping away from work for a season. It wasn't easy, but for me, it was necessary. Dale and I made that decision together to protect my strength and allow my body the time and space it needed to recover.

That didn't mean withdrawing from life. It meant making changes that supported recovery. Each person's journey will look different, but the goal is the same: listen to the body, seek peace, and choose calm over constant pressure.

Connecting the Dots

The evidence revealed that my battle with cancer was deeply connected to a weakened immune system. And as I continued to learn, a simple but powerful truth became apparent.

Cancer cannot exist in a body with a strong immune system.

In the following chapters, we move to the other side of the journey where real transformation occurs. This is where we begin restoring strength, rebuilding health, and discovering the keys to winning the battle against cancer.

Chapter 10

The Secret Weapon

Many people search for a single solution. A magic bullet that will restore their health. Yet the most powerful tool for healing has been within the body all along: the immune system.

Its miraculous design enables it to recognize threats, repair damage, and defend the body against disease. When we learn to support and strengthen this system, we activate one of the body's greatest resources for healing.

Healing can begin at any point—when damage is reduced, and the body is given what it needs to repair itself, renew damaged cells, and restore balance naturally.

In simple terms, the immune system is a remarkable, around-the-clock defense network. It's made up of specialized cells, tissues, and organs that work together to protect the body from harm caused by germs, toxins, bacteria, viruses, and damaged cells.

One of its most important roles is knowing the difference between what belongs in the body and what doesn't. The immune system recognizes your healthy cells as "self," and identifies harmful invaders as "non-self." Then, it goes to work removing threats and clearing damaged cells, helping your body stay strong and well.

A medical doctor who had overcome her own cancer naturally—without chemotherapy or radiation—shared a truth that changed the way I understood healing from cancer.

She looked at me with complete confidence and said, "Paula, you wouldn't have cancer if your immune system were working properly."

Her words stopped me in my tracks.

Cancer would never have taken hold in my body if my immune system had been healthy.

After three more days of research, I understood her words were true. Once again, what I believed about cancer and my health shifted.

Was it really that simple?

My mission became unmistakable: rebuild my immune system as quickly as possible. If there is such a thing as a magic bullet against cancer or other health issues, this was it.

A strong immune system.

The more I learned, the clearer things became. Caring for my body's health had always been a personal responsibility. But it had taken an extreme health crisis for me to realize it.

For me, learning what to do wasn't the hard part. The real challenge was putting it into practice—that took focus and commitment.

My lifestyle had weakened my natural defenses and disrupted the very part of me meant to protect. But once the cause became clear, the solution was even clearer.

From that day forward, every decision came down to one question. A question that I asked myself every day, all day, about everything—

Will This Weaken or Strengthen My Immune System?

The answer to that one question led to immediate changes. Toxic inputs and harmful habits had to stop. Now.

It was time to restore what the body needed.

Nutrients. Pure water. Vitamins. Minerals. Peace instead of stress. And adequate rest.

The Powerhouse Protector

The immune system is the powerhouse God created to heal our bodies. Every person has one. When a finger is cut, or a cold virus shows up, it is the immune system that responds—repairing tissue, fighting infection, and restoring healthy balance.

The truth of the situation was becoming extremely clear: Cancer would not be in my body if I had a strong immune system. Yet in today's toxic and often uninformed culture, few people understand how to protect their health by caring for this incredible system. I certainly didn't before my diagnosis.

The immune system is our body's most important defense against sickness and disease.

Imagine a military unit that's assigned to protect you. But their food is poisoned. Their water is contaminated and scarce. Explosions surround their camp, causing continual anxiety. Soon, they are weak, exhausted, and overwhelmed.

That's what happens to the immune system when the body is bombarded with toxins, dehydration, and chronic stress.

When I chose to take responsibility for strengthening my immune system, I regained a sense of control over the cancer that threatened me.

Understanding that cancer cannot thrive in a body supported by a strong immune system was shocking. Could it really be that logical? Was it as understandable as cause-and-effect? Yes, I believed it was!

Back to the Basics

When pausing to ask whether the food was *God-created* or *man-made*, it became surprisingly easy to determine whether it was a healthy choice for my body.

Healing naturally is a process—it takes time. Time was something the doctor said I had very little of. The doctor's plan was more surgery, aggressive chemo, radiation, and drugs, if I wanted to live longer than six months.

However, in my research, there was documented evidence that both chemotherapy and radiation are known to potentially cause cancer. This knowledge stirred a question: how could using a treatment that can cause cancer help me get rid of cancer? That made no sense.

The more I researched the doctor's prescribed course of action, the clearer my path became. My guiding truth for every decision was whether it would help or hurt my immune system. Ultimately, my response to the treatments was a hard "No." My resistance brought friction between the medical protocol and myself, creating an impasse. I never returned.

My doctor was doing what doctors are trained to do —focus on removing and treating the symptoms of cancer.

But no longer did I feel led to participate in *symptom treatment*. Solving the root cause of cancer had become my focused goal.

The real issue was deeper than a tumor. My immune system itself needed to recover its health and become strong enough to do the work it was created to do.

Honoring God's Design

Of the three parts of every person—body, soul, and spirit, the body is often the easiest to understand. It is the part we can see and touch.

It's what allows us to see, hear, move, feel, and engage with the world around us. So, when illness appears, it often shows up first in the body.

Before learning the information I'm sharing with you, a health problem usually meant a visit to the doctor.

Please understand, there is deep gratitude for the doctors who walked alongside me during the early days of cancer. At the same time, it became clear early on that managing my own health was a personal responsibility—one that requires daily participation.

Effective healing often involves multiple pathways. At times, God does work through the medical industry. But more often, He works through the natural resources He has already provided. Things like nutrient-rich food, herbs, clean water, rest, stress reduction, emotional support, and disciplined daily decisions.

Healing naturally from cancer involves education, renewed thinking... and time. Learning how God designed the body to function offers a starting point—one that's both practical and empowering. It doesn't have to be complicated. In fact, it's a path of common sense.

The information provided in this book can offer helpful insight, but there's no one-size-fits-all formula. Reliable principles of health and healing, both natural and spiritual, can offer guidance. Yet every journey is unique because every life and situation is unique.

That's why I can say this:

Once you understand how the body is designed to operate and the principles of lasting health, you become the most qualified person to take charge of guiding your health journey.

Supporting the Immune System

Diet became a central part of my healing process. My body needed nutrient-rich support to help recover and regain strength.

My approach was extreme by most standards. But I was fully engaged. I knew that half measures would not serve me well. According to my doctor, I had very little time to turn things around.

The threat was real, and I wanted to live. I decided to act in faith and fight as though my life depended on it—because it did.

Scripture offers wisdom for every part of life, including the daily choices that shape our health. One verse that speaks clearly to this is:

"Therefore, whether you eat or drink, or whatever you do, do all to the glory of God."

—1 Corinthians 10:31.

Once the connection between diet and immune health became clear, strengthening my immune system became a priority. What I ate and drank was not only important to my health—it was also something within my control.

A Season of Discipline

A strict diet during my battle with cancer was for a season. I approached it with serious discipline because my desire to live was powerful and motivating. There were certainly moments of temptation, but life was too precious to compromise. I knew this was something that needed to be done correctly the first time.

Each person reading this may choose a different level of discipline, and those choices are personal. The aggressive diet I followed lasted about eighteen months. After that, foods like birthday cake or the occasional juicy steak gradually returned—but in moderation. Paying attention to what I ate and drank became a conscious part of supporting and maintaining a strong immune system.

The Dietary Approach I Chose

One of my first food changes was eliminating all animal products—including meat and dairy. This provided a clean foundation for healing and helped create a more alkaline internal environment in my body.

It became clear that certain foods and beverages placed added stress on my already weakened system, while others helped create conditions where healing could thrive.

Breaking a long-standing habit with caffeine wasn't easy. But a cancer diagnosis has a way of clarifying priorities. Every choice mattered.

Suddenly, meals became simple and plant-based. Organic foods took center stage, foods like fresh salads, soups, vegetables, fruits, nuts, beans, and seeds. Whole foods, such as organic whole-grain oatmeal, became a steady part of my daily nourishment.

Juicing organic vegetables became one of my primary healing practices. It proved to be so important that I'll share more about it in the next chapter.

My focus was simple: nutrient-dense foods, pure water, managing stress, getting enough rest, and renewing my mind and spirit each day through Scripture. This included speaking healing affirmations aloud. Somedays, multiple times. These were not extreme measures. They were basic, powerful choices meant to help my whole person move toward restoration instead of resistance.

Local raw honey became an occasional sweetener. Unsweetened almond or oat milk became dairy alternatives, which I used minimally, ultimately preferring coconut milk.

Soy was avoided, since much of the conventional supply is genetically modified and heavily processed. My focus remained on reducing chemical exposure and the issues with processed foods. I continued to make choices that supported my body with foods that I kept as close to their natural state as possible.

Additional Immune Boosting Techniques

To further support my immune strength, I added several key supplements. Daily high-quality multivitamins, minerals, antioxidants, organic green barley caplets, Vitamin D, B12, and B17. I took Vitamin C —2,000 mg in the morning and another 2,000 mg in the afternoon, with food. Together, these choices became a daily ritual.

As I've said repeatedly, God designed the human body with a remarkable ability to heal. It was meant to be nourished by natural, whole, life-giving foods. For that reason, I avoided processed and artificial foods completely. They offer little nourishment and only add stress to the body.

For me, healing began with awareness. From there, it grew through simple, intentional choices. As I learned healthier habits and began choosing cleaner foods and drinks, my body started to respond. I felt stronger and more resilient. Little by little, my body was changing, and my immune system was becoming stronger and better able to function the way it was designed to.

No matter where you start on your own healing journey, you can move forward with confidence. Every step you take toward health is important. I'm speaking from my own experience, but I believe many people will discover the same thing I did. When you support your body and strengthen your immune system, your health will begin to improve again. Healing can return.

I often remind myself that God created my body not only to survive, but also to heal from sickness or injury. Lasting health and healing from cancer are not only possible—they are part of God's design for the human body.

Healing Starts in the Mind

One additional and important area of restored and lasting health deserves attention before moving on: attitude and thoughts.

When the mind and attitude do not align with healing, a powerful part of the body, soul, and spirit's ability to recover is left unused.

In my case, learning to see myself as healed—despite symptoms and fear—was essential. Believing and acting as though healing was already at work and already belonged to me opened doors that reached deeply into my spirit and soul, putting me in a receiving mode.

Another area I quickly recognized, was my perspective on whether I was the "victim" or the "victor." I realized that I could not identify as a cancer patient or even a person with cancer. It was imperative that I identify as a healed, healthy, and well person first.

The Bible taught me some valuable lessons about faith. Faith always identifies with the answer first, before the answer comes. I knew this battle would be no different. Again, it was about choices. I choose not to tell people, "I had cancer." Or to talk about my symptoms. Words are powerful, and I wanted mine to work toward my healing, not against me.

The Bible describes this approach as *faith (to learn about real faith and how it works, especially for healing, I recommend reading the book:* Atomic Faith*)*.

Throughout my battle, as I included my deeper understanding of faith, my whole person—body, soul, and spirit—was able to participate more fully and powerfully in the process.

As we continue this journey together, there is still more to uncover and apply. Let's continue building on what's been shared and move even closer to lasting health and freedom from cancer.

Chapter 11

The Juice Advantage

Fresh organic vegetable juice was a central part of my health recovery. The reason juicing mattered so much and became my primary protocol is due to its ability to rapidly rebuild immune strength. Juicing was the most aggressive, natural, proactive step I could take.

(This topic can be explored in greater detail in *the Winning Over Cancer Coaching Video Program,* including demonstration, recipes, and practical guidance.)

As I mentioned earlier, my immune system had been depleted. It had weakened until it no longer protected my body. I believe this was the primary reason cancer was able to take hold and grow.

My cells needed nutrient-rich nourishment. And they needed it quickly. My goal was clear—to rebuild my body's natural defenses against disease by rebuilding my immune system.

Fresh organic juice delivers a concentrated supply of nutrients in a form the body can absorb quickly. In my case, it was one of the fastest ways to restore what my body had been lacking.

Juicing provides concentrated, natural vitamins, minerals, and beneficial plant compounds—including living enzymes—without placing added strain on digestion. It became a powerful, yet gentle way to support my body's health and restore balance.

Juicing is a natural remedy that I consider God's medicine for my body. But timing is crucial for effectiveness.

Guidance for Juicing

Fresh organic vegetable juice—when consumed on an empty stomach—rapidly absorbs into the bloodstream in as little as twenty minutes. This transfers concentrated nutrients throughout the body, quickly nourishing cells, supporting repair, and strengthening the immune system.

If solid foods such as fruits or vegetables are eaten first, waiting about forty minutes usually gives the stomach enough time to empty before drinking fresh juice.

However, if juice is consumed *with* solid food, the body directs it through the digestive system. This redirects both delays and minimizes the amount of nutrients that reach the cells.

In addition, when juice is added to a stomach still working on solids, digestion slows, fermentation can occur, and much of the juice's healing potential is lost.

Juicing on an empty stomach is powerful, delivering nutrients quickly into the bloodstream to strengthen the immune system.

Buying organic vegetables and taking the time to juice were significant investments in my health. So, it didn't make sense to compromise the benefits by mixing juice with any solid food.

Vegetables vs Fruit

An important distinction emerged between juicing vegetables and juicing fruit. Vegetable juice provides concentrated vitamins, minerals, enzymes, and phytonutrients with minimal impact on blood sugar. Fruit, however, contains natural sugars that are normally balanced by fiber when eaten raw.

Once fruit is juiced, that fiber is removed, allowing sugar to enter the bloodstream rapidly. This can spike blood sugar and insulin levels and add stress on the body at a time when it needs calm and healing support.

For these reasons, the focus remained primarily on juicing organic vegetables. Fruit, when eaten, was consumed raw, so the fiber remained intact. Fruit juice was avoided altogether. This approach provided powerful nutrition without overwhelming the system, keeping the emphasis on steady healing rather than quick energy.

The early days of juicing began with a simple combination of organic carrots and an apple. Carrots contain valuable plant compounds, including beta-carotene and other antioxidants, that have been studied for their potential to support cellular health. Carrots also contain compounds that researchers believe may have anti-carcinogenic (cancer-fighting) properties.

Apples are the only fruit that can be combined with vegetables without a downside. They tend to blend well without raising concerns, unlike some other fruits. They also add natural sweetness, along with vitamin C and other helpful nutrients.

Organic Benefits

Due to the much higher nutrient content of organic produce and the absence of potentially toxic pesticides, I chose, whenever possible, to juice and eat organic produce.

Using organic produce also allowed me to sidestep dangerous toxins like glyphosate, a widely used herbicide (weed killer), that often leaves residue on non-organic fruits and vegetables.

Occasionally, when organic wasn't available or affordable, I used non-organic vegetables and washed them carefully with a spray wash for produce to reduce toxic residues. However, organic produce was always my first choice.

Once juicing became familiar and my routine felt stable, I branched out by adding other ingredients to my carrot-apple juice. Organic beets, celery, spinach, cucumber, ginger, kale, collards, romaine, parsley, etc., which expanded the range of nutrients and flavors and supported my body in additional ways. But the carrot-apple remained my daily staple.

Drinking in Nature's Healing

An 8 oz. glass of organic juice every 1½ to 2 hours provided steady nourishment throughout the day. This regular rhythm of intake seemed most effective—like a dose of natural medicine.

When juicing was spaced throughout the day, the body appeared to benefit more readily than when larger amounts were taken only a few times a day.

Because fresh nutrients and enzymes are living and delicate, prolonged exposure to air weakens their potency. Any juice saved for later was stored in sealed glass quart jars in the refrigerator.

Juicing Routine

My routine was to prepare fresh juice twice daily—once in the morning and again in the afternoon. This maintained a steady supply, which was refrigerated until needed. When away from home, a quart jar in a small cooler made it possible to continue having regular servings.

Juicing was never about rigid rules. It was about providing the body with steady nutritional support. Typically, eight to ten glasses of fresh, organic vegetable juice were consumed each day, beginning first thing in the morning, continuing every couple of hours throughout the day, and ending with a final serving shortly before bed.

Understanding how the body absorbs nutrients helped me see that juicing could be a precise and powerful tool for healing. And I was committed to utilizing its benefits.

pH Balance: Why It Matters for Healing

As my understanding of how the body functions deepened, the importance of pH balance became increasingly clear. At first, I'll admit, it sounded a little intimidating—almost like chemistry class all over again. But the more I learned, the simpler it became.

I discovered that the body's internal environment is usually either acidic or alkaline.

On the pH scale, zero represents extreme acidity, fourteen depicts extreme alkalinity, and seven is neutral.

Research suggests that healthy cells function best in a more alkaline environment. Plant-based foods naturally help create alkalinity in the body, reinforcing the value of choosing foods that support healing. What fascinated me was how much our daily choices influence that internal environment.

Have you ever noticed how different you feel after eating fresh fruits and vegetables for several days compared to eating heavily processed foods? The body notices the difference, too.

Instead of constantly asking, "What can I eat?" I began asking a different question:

"What environment am I creating inside my body every single day?"

That question changed the way I looked at food.

On the other hand, animal products create a more acidic environment in the body, which is more supportive of cancer cell growth. This knowledge made maintaining a more alkaline internal balance desirable.

In the end, pH wasn't something I worried about, and here's why. Gradually and naturally, my body became more alkaline automatically. Because of my juicing and largely plant-based practices, my pH adjusted itself naturally. My pH reflected the healthier choices I was making each day.

Healing involved more than juicing and diet. Practical, everyday habits also became important in supporting the body's natural ability to recover. Simple health practices worked together to strengthen and support the body throughout the healing process.

Rest: The Natural Reset

Adequate rest became a vital part of my victory over cancer. I learned that the body repairs and restores itself most effectively during deep, consistent sleep. And the immune system requires rest to recharge and function at its best.

The human body is designed to follow a natural rhythm known as the circadian cycle, a pattern shaped by light and darkness, day and night. When this rhythm is honored, the body is better able to regulate hormones, manage stress, and maintain internal balance.

My sleep began to improve little by little. Very quickly, I gave up my alarm clock. For the first time since childhood, I allowed my body to wake naturally when it felt rested. For me, that was a remarkable change.

For many years, I had sacrificed rest in the name of productivity. Through this healing journey, something important became clear to me: rest is not a luxury. It is during rest that the body does some of its deepest healing.

Oxygen: Fuel for Cellular Healing

I discovered that oxygen plays a vital role in cellular health. Healthy cells depend on a steady oxygen supply to function properly and maintain strength. Breathing, movement, and environment influence how well oxygen circulates through the body and supplies the cells.

Activity gradually increased through gentle exercise, especially daily walks when strength allowed. Movement improved circulation and supported overall well-being.

My breathing also became more intentional. On days when exercise wasn't possible, I focused on taking slow, deep breaths throughout the day to keep oxygen circulating. Time outdoors in fresh air was welcomed whenever possible. And open windows brought that same freshness inside.

Simple practices—deep breathing, fresh air, gentle movement, and exercise—became meaningful parts of the healing process. In time, their impact contributed to my complete healing.

Water: A Simple, Yet Essential Healing Tool

Water is essential to nearly every function in the body. It supports circulation, digestion, detoxification, nutrient transport, and cellular health. All of this is vital to healing and immune strength.

Although the body is made largely of water, many people live in a state of chronic dehydration. I certainly had.

Even mild dehydration can place stress on the body, contributing to fatigue, poor circulation, and inflammation. Understanding this helped make proper hydration a daily priority.

It also became obvious that not all water is equal. Tap and basic filtered water may still contain additives such as fluoride, while some bottled waters have been shown to contain microplastics and other unwanted contaminants. With an already strained immune system, choosing clean, well-filtered water became important to my healing journey.

Proper hydration helps the body function more efficiently. It supports the body's natural ability to cleanse, repair, and restore itself. Over time, it became clear to me that when the body lacks quality water, every system must work harder.

Staying well hydrated proved to be a simple but powerful foundation for my healing. Drinking enough clean water every day strengthened every other step I was taking.

One helpful hydration guideline is: drink about **half your body weight in ounces of water each day**. For example, someone who weighs 150 pounds would aim for about 75 ounces daily. Of course, individual needs can vary, but this guideline provided a helpful starting point.

For me, proper hydration became one more simple daily habit that helped my body move steadily back toward health. A nuance of hydration for me was sipping consistently throughout the day rather than taking in larger servings of water only a few times.

As I began caring for my whole person—body, soul, and spirit—bringing each part back into harmony, something started to change.

My once sick and cancer-filled body responded.

Strength returned. Balance followed. Healing was taking place—steadily, day by day.

After eighteen long months of standing in faith... making the changes in my lifestyle that I have shared with you—

Declaring truth even when I could not yet see it—

Realigning my body with the way it was created to function—

Allowing healing to flow from heaven into my life through faith—

Finally...

The cancer was gone.

Completely gone.

My health was gradually, quietly restored—without chemotherapy, without radiation, and without drugs or more surgery.

That was over twenty-five years ago.

One of the great benefits of learning how to help my body heal is the confidence that comes from understanding how to care for my health.

Not once since... have I lived with the fear of cancer returning.

Because this was not just a moment of "healing" for me, it became a new way of living. And although the extreme diet is no longer part of daily life, being mindful of how my health is managed has remained an ongoing priority.

As my body, soul, and spirit began to function more in harmony with the way they were designed, healing became more than something to be hoped for occasionally.

It became a continual reality.

Not temporary.

But a way of life.

Chapter 12

From My Heart to Yours

As this book ends, I want to thank you for walking through this deeply personal journey with me.

My prayer is that somewhere within these pages, you discovered truths, insights, and encouragement that helped you find your own path forward—one step at a time. Whether you are personally facing cancer, walking beside someone you love, or simply searching for answers, I pray this book reminds you that there is hope, there is wisdom to be found, and there can still be life and health on the other side of cancer.

When I was first diagnosed, I admit, I panicked. A diagnosis like cancer can make a person feel as though their whole world has suddenly stopped. At the same time, others expected me to take quick, decisive action even before I understood what my options were.

One of the greatest lessons I trust you take from this

book is that there is no need to panic. There is time to become educated. Time to better understand what is happening in your body. Time to carefully consider your options and make informed choices about the path ahead.

Whatever the challenges you face, I encourage you never to lose sight of the God who created your body with an incredible ability to heal and restore.

There is something very relevant at a time when cancer strikes. It is the fear of losing life. Every person on the planet will experience both life and death. Neither are avoidable. Currently, you are experiencing life. And whether through sickness, an accident, or simply the passing of time, death is a reality you and every other person will face.

Your life is precious, and no one else has the right to decide what you do at a time when you are dealing with a disease like cancer. Only you. The decisions ahead are life-or-death choices. So, taking the time to make each choice with wisdom is the gift you can give yourself.

Early in my journey, I made sure my relationship with God was where it needed to be. Honestly, I believe that matters for every person, not only during sickness, but throughout life itself.

What I discovered was a loving Father who cared deeply about me, even amid uncertainty. I found peace in knowing that God loved me and wanted me well. However, that peace did not remove the challenges ahead. But it changed how I walked through them and who walked through them with me. It wasn't something I had to face alone.

If there is one final message I hope reaches your heart, it is this: you are deeply valuable. Your life matters. God loves you, cares for you, and desires wholeness and life for you.

No matter what report you may have received or what fears may stand before you, God has made a way toward life, healing, peace, and restoration. And as you continue to seek Him, ask for His wisdom, and follow His leading, He is faithful to guide you toward the help, understanding, and direction you need for the journey ahead.

In my own case, I came back to the understanding that my life belongs to God. I realized again that Jesus Christ is the Savior I need and truly, the Savior every person needs. I also chose to make Jesus the Lord of my life. That decision is one of the reasons I am alive today. He faithfully led me to the truths I needed and gave me wisdom to make changes that restored my health because He is a God of life and love.

My belief is not in religion or any specific church. It is in a personal relationship with Jesus.

If you are unsure of your relationship with God and

would like to know with certainty that Jesus is your Savior, I invite you to visit my website and click on *Meet Jesus*. There is a personal video message just for you that will help you establish a personal relationship with God through Jesus Christ. I hope you will take a few moments to watch it.

I am not trying to present myself as someone who has all the answers. I am simply sharing what helped me, what strengthened me, and what gave me guidance when I desperately needed it.

In the next few pages, I've included a brief recap of the **10 Facts I wish I Knew Before Being Diagnosed**. As you read through them, I trust that these truths will settle deeply into your heart and mind, just as they eventually did mine.

There is certainly much more that could be said. There is not enough room in one small book to share everything I learned throughout my journey. But I truly believe what you have read here is enough to help you begin, enough to help you move forward with greater wisdom, greater peace, and greater faith.

Begin turning your attention toward the solution. In my own life, I found that fear weakened me, but faith strengthened me.

I also learned how important it is to support and rebuild the incredible body God designed—especially the immune system.

Please also take a moment to look at the valuable

Free Gift I've included for you in the following pages. I believe it will encourage and help you continue moving forward.

During one of the hardest seasons of my life, the Lord brought me to a Scripture promise that became an anchor for my soul. I held onto it then, and I still hold onto it today. Hopefully, it will encourage you.

"God is faithful, who will not allow you to be tempted beyond what you are able, but with the temptation will also make the way of escape..." —1 Corinthians 10:13

That promise reminded me that God always has a way forward, even when we cannot yet see it.

Thank you again for allowing me to share part of my story with you, along with some of the information I wish I had known when I was first diagnosed.

Please know that I am praying for you. I believe good things are ahead for you. No matter what your present circumstances may look like, remember that your story is not over.

Take one step at a time. Keep your eyes on God and His promises. Continue learning. Continue believing. Continue moving forward with faith for healing.

And always remember:

"It is the truth that makes us free."

With love and prayers,

Paula

Appendix A

10 Facts I Wish I Knew Before Being Diagnosed

1. You have time, and there are options.
2. Educate before you commit to a path.
3. Cancer is the result of cause-and-effect.
4. Facts are not always the truth.
5. The tumor is not the cancer.
6. Cancer is not a foreign invader—it is our own damaged cells.
7. Cancer is a systemic disease—the entire system is sick.
8. Cancer cannot take hold in a body with a strong immune system.
9. Both chemo and radiation treatments are known to cause cancer and weaken the immune system.

10. Medical treatments manage symptoms of cancer, while often making the root problem worse.

The 10 Facts Explained

1. You have time, and there are options.

If you or someone you love is facing cancer, it's important to know that you have time. There is time to process, learn, and make informed choices that are based on truth, not panic. What you do *first* can greatly shape everything that follows.

2. Educate yourself before you commit to a path.

Cancer doesn't arrive in the body randomly. There are often underlying conditions, imbalances, deficiencies, stress, toxicity, or weaknesses that develop over time and create an environment in which disease can grow. One of the most important things to do is: slow down and become educated before committing to any path.

By learning what is true, you can make thoughtful, informed choices instead of emotional ones. Truth matters. Facts can be faulty. And it is the understanding of truth that helps us to make wiser choices that support life and healing.

3. Cancer is the result of cause-and-effect.

Where you see an *effect*, such as cancer or another disease, there is an underlying *cause*. Most health problems do not appear overnight but develop over time due to accumulated factors.

One of the most important steps is taking time to identify what may have contributed to your personal condition in the first place, because understanding the cause often reveals the path toward healing.

4. Facts are not always the truth.

Facts can change, but truth does not. Facts are often based on current observations, limited understanding, or human interpretation, which means they can change as new information is discovered or a consensus is revised.

But the truth is constant. It never changes. Truth does not shift with opinions, circumstances, or time.

Truth is real, reliable, and anchored in something immovable.

5. The tumor is not the cancer.

A medical doctor once pulled me aside and explained that the tumor was not the entirety of the cancer—it was a visible symptom of a deeper problem taking place within the body. The tumor was evidence that cancer did exist, but it also served as a warning sign that something more significant was happening beneath the surface. That understanding helped me realize I needed to better understand and address the underlying conditions within my body that had allowed cancer to develop and grow. Because if I only removed the tumor, without addressing the deeper problem, it would simply grow back again.

6. Cancer is not a foreign invader—it's our own damaged cells.

When first diagnosed, I assumed I was just one of the unlucky ones—still believing that cancer was random and it had unfortunately landed on me. But I discovered that cancer was made up of my own cells that had become damaged. Learning what was causing my cells to become damaged was a step toward making changes to regain my health.

7. Cancer is a systemic disease—the entire system is sick.

I finally understood that cancer is a systemic disease—meaning the entire system in the body is weak and sick. Knowing the truth about cancer, I realized that if I didn't treat the root cause of my problem, more tumors would be the result. The tumors were real and malignant. But the tumors were only a physical indication of the unhealthiness of my entire system. Eliminating the tumor was like cutting off a weed at ground level, while leaving the roots intact to grow a new weed.

8. Cancer cannot grow if there is a strong immune system.

Abnormal or damaged cells occur in every person's body. The difference lies in the individual's immune system health. Most have an immune system that captures and eliminates damaged cells, removing them from the body. However, if the immune system is weak and the source of the damage persists or worsens, the immune system becomes less able to control abnormal cell growth. If that occurs, the problem escalates into a fully compromised system that allows cancer to multiply.

9. Chemo and radiation treatments are known to cause cancer, while they weaken the immune system.

Chemo and radiation treatments are a double-edged sword. They do kill and shrink fast-growing cancer cells, but at the same time, they can kill healthy cells and cause cancer in a percentage of the people exposed. These protocols also damage other tissues and organs in the body that are subjected to the treatment. The boundary for me was that both of these treatments further damage and weaken the all-important immune system. Once I turned my focus to correcting the root problem—which was a weak immune system—these treatments were no longer on my radar.

10. Medical treatments manage symptoms of cancer, while often making the root problem worse.

My battle through cancer is written in detail in my book *"Life, Cancer and God."* What I am sharing in this book is basic and limited. The goal here is to give you some essential truths to help you take your first steps through the process. However, as I learned more about the cancer industry and the protocols for treating cancer, it became clear that their methods are exclusive to managing the *symptoms* of cancer, not treating the root cause. Once I learned how and why I got cancer...

and I learned that my body was designed to heal disease if I had a strong immune system, my focus shifted from the problem to the solution. I committed to naturally rebuilding my immune system as quickly and effectively as possible.

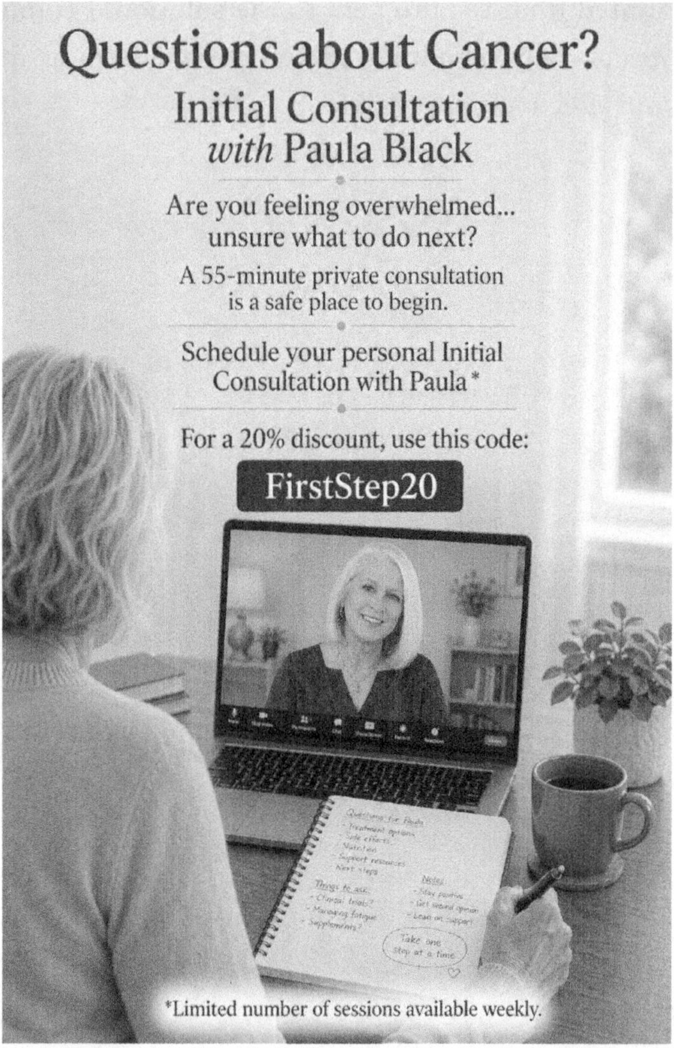
Questions about Cancer?
Initial Consultation
with Paula Black
Are you feeling overwhelmed...
unsure what to do next?
A 55-minute private consultation
is a safe place to begin.
Schedule your personal Initial
Consultation with Paula*
For a 20% discount, use this code:
FirstStep20
*Limited number of sessions available weekly.

APPENDIX B

Healing and Faith Scriptures & Affirmations

Healing and Faith Scriptures

(Scriptures are New King James & Amplified Bible)

The Word of God will save your life.

"My son, give attention to my words; incline your ear to my sayings. Do not let them depart from your eyes; keep them in the midst of your heart; for they are life to those who find them, and health to all their flesh. Keep your heart with all diligence, for out of it spring the issues of life."

Proverbs 4:20-23 (NKJV)

God's benefits include healing.

"Bless the Lord, O my soul; and all that is within me, bless His holy name! Bless the Lord, O my soul, And forget not all His benefits; Who forgives all your iniquities, Who heals all your diseases, Who redeems your life from destruction, Who crowns you with loving kindness and tender mercies, Who satisfies your mouth with good things, so that your youth is renewed like the eagle's."

Psalm 103:1-5 (NKJV)

God's Word will not fail, and you can establish your faith in it.

"...Man shall not live and be upheld and sustained by bread alone, but by every word that comes forth from the mouth of God."

Matthew 4:4 (NKJV)

"But the Word of the Lord (divine instruction, the Gospel) endures forever, and this Word is the good news which was preached to you."

1 Peter 1:25 (AMP)

"Roll your works upon the Lord [commit and trust them wholly to Him; He will cause your thoughts to become agreeable to His will, and] so shall your plans be established and succeed."

Proverbs 16:3 (AMP)

Cast down thoughts and imaginations that don't line up with the word of God.

"For the weapons of our warfare are not carnal but mighty in God for pulling down strongholds, casting down arguments and every high thing that exalts itself against the knowledge of God, bringing every thought into captivity to the obedience of Christ."

2 Corinthians 10:4-5 (NKJV)

Your choice matters.

"I call heaven and earth to witness this day against you that I have set before you life and death, the blessings and the curses; therefore choose life, that you and your descendants may live."

Deuteronomy 30:19 (NKJV)

What you "believe" matters.

"Therefore I say to you, whatever things you ask when you pray, **believe** that you receive them, and you will have them."

Mark 11:24 (NKJV)

God's Word is healing.

"He sent His word and healed them, and delivered them from their destructions."

Psalm 107:20 (NKJV)

Fear is not from God... Faith overpowers it!

"For God has not given us a spirit of fear, but of power and of love and of a sound mind."

2 Timothy 1:7 (NKJV)

Establish faith for your healing.

"So faith comes by hearing [what is told], and hearing by the Word (rhema) of God."

Romans 10:17 (AMP)

What is faith?

"Now Faith is the assurance (the confirmation, the title deed) of things hoped for, the proof of things we do not see."

Hebrews 11:1 (AMP)

We live by faith.

"For we walk by faith, not by sight."

2 Corinthians 5:7 (NKJV)

Have the elders of your church pray for your healing. (If they believe in healing and follow the instructions in the Bible.)

"Is anyone among you sick? He should call in the church elders (the spiritual guides), and they should pray over him, anointing him with oil in the Lord's name."

James 5:14 (AMP)

God promises His children a long life.

"With long life I will satisfy him, and show him my salvation."

Psalm 91:16 (NKJV)

Jesus bore your sins and your sickness.

"Surely He has borne our griefs (sickness, weakness, and distresses) and carried our sorrows and pains [of punishment] yet we ignorantly considered Him stricken, smitten and afflicted by God. But He was wounded for our transgressions, He was bruised for our iniquities; the chastisement of our peace was upon Him, and by His stripes we are healed."

Isaiah 53:4-5 (AMP)

Establish faith for your healing.

"So faith comes by hearing [what is told], and hearing by the Word (rhema) of God."

Romans 10:17 (AMP)

God wants you to live.

"I shall not die, but live, and declare the works of the Lord."

Psalm 118:17 (NKJV)

You must take authority over the sickness in your body.

"Assuredly, I say to you, whatever you bind on earth will be bound in heaven, and whatever you loose on earth will be loosed in heaven."

Matthew 18:18 (NKJV)

Agree with someone for your healing.

"Again I say to you that if two of you agree on earth concerning anything that they ask, it will be done for them by My Father in heaven."

Matthew 18:19 (NKJV)

What you "say" matters.

"So Jesus answered and said to them, "Have faith in God. For assuredly I say to you, whoever **says** to this mountain, 'Be removed and be cast into the sea,' and does not doubt in his heart, but **believes** that those things he **says** will come to pass, he will have whatever he **says**."

Mark 11:22-23 (NKJV)

Fear is not from God... build your faith!

"For God has not given us a spirit of fear, but of power and of love and of a sound mind."

2 Timothy 1:7 (NKJV)

We can have confidence.

"And this is the confidence (the assurance, the privilege of boldness), which we have in Him; that if we ask anything according to His will (in agreement with His own plan), He listens to and hears us. And if we [positively] know that He listens to us in whatever we ask, we also know [with settled and absolute knowledge] that we have [granted us as our present possessions] the request made of Him."

1 John 5:14-15 (AMP)

We cannot please God without faith.

"But without faith it is impossible to please Him, for he who comes to God must believe that He is, and that He is a rewarder of those who diligently seek Him."

Hebrews 11:6 (NKJV)

Affirmations

Affirmations are like proclamations. You speak what you desire for your future. These affirmations align you with life and health, not death and sickness. What you don't say is just as important as what you say.

Words are vessels of power—to create and build up, or damage and destroy.

During my battle with cancer, once I knew God's will for my situation, I committed my course through bringing my words and actions into agreement with what I believed.

From that time on, I never spoke again about being sick, having cancer, or that I might die. I only spoke what I believed was God's will for me—healing and life.

That doesn't mean negative, fearful thoughts never entered my mind—in fact, they plagued my mind regularly. But I had made a choice. I knew I could not walk or speak in faith *and* doubt at the same time, and still get the result I was believing for.

My Scriptures and affirmations kept my faith strong and my goals focused on getting well and living a long life.

Ephesians 6:13 in the Amplified translation: *"Therefore put on God's complete armor, that you may be able to resist and stand your ground on the evil day [of danger], and, having done all [the crisis demands], to stand [firmly in your place]."*

I was going to stand firm and do all I could do—for as long as it took.

It's important to understand that affirmations, or proclamations of faith, don't change God—He never changes. It is always His will for you to be healed.

But they do change you. Continuously speaking words of faith helps you stay in agreement with God and is an act of faith.

Here are some principles I follow when speaking affirmations:

I always speak affirmations out loud in the present tense as if what I believe already exists—I perceive my desired outcome as being real now.

My affirmations are always positive, not negative.

I try to keep the affirmations short so I can focus my faith with strong conviction and clear thought on what I am saying.

When I speak my affirmations, I speak with force and confidence—releasing my faith through my words.

I use faith to fight fear, and I use my affirmations the same way. If I am feeling fearful or doubtful, I repeat the affirmations—alone, aloud, and with confident force. I always speak them out loud at least once every day. More often if needed.

Adjust them to fit your personal situation, but be sure to keep them in agreement with God's Word.

Here are examples of affirmations I used when I had cancer:

I repent for any actions that damaged my health, and I'm working with God to bring healing and life back into my body.

I am a child of God, and His promises are true.

God loves me, and He has given me a future and a hope.

I am a partner with God to accomplish His will in my life.

I am healed because of what Jesus did for me.

I give God full authority over my life—body, soul, and spirit.

I am healed according to God's Word.

I recognize and accept the excellence of my healing plan. Cancer has no authority to remain in my body.

My body is a gift from God and the temple of the Holy Spirit.

I am helping my body heal each day by managing my health.

I enjoy eating healthy foods that God created... and I enjoy how healthy foods make me feel.

I'm a faithful steward of the body God has given me.

I live every day in gratitude and forgiveness.

My faith is strong because I hear God's Word spoken and I believe it.

With God's help, nothing is too hard for me.

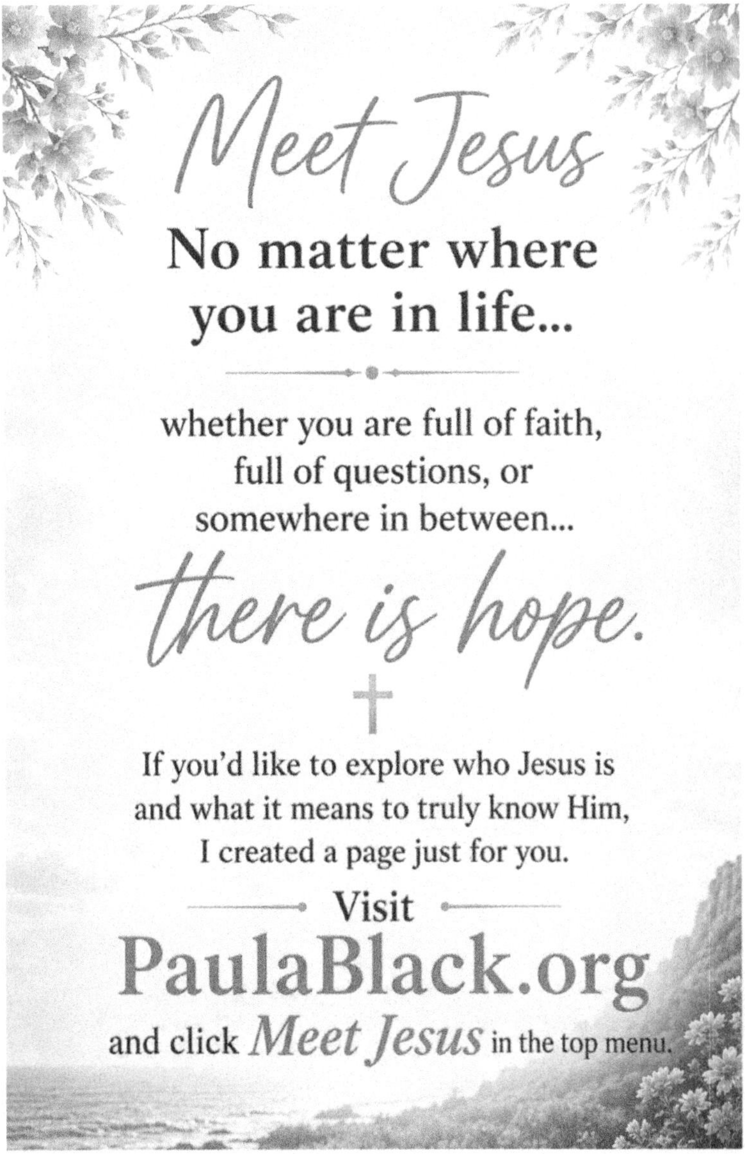
Meet Jesus
No matter where
you are in life...
whether you are full of faith,
full of questions, or
somewhere in between...
there is hope.
If you'd like to explore who Jesus is
and what it means to truly know Him,
I created a page just for you.
Visit
PaulaBlack.org
and click Meet Jesus in the top menu.

About the Author

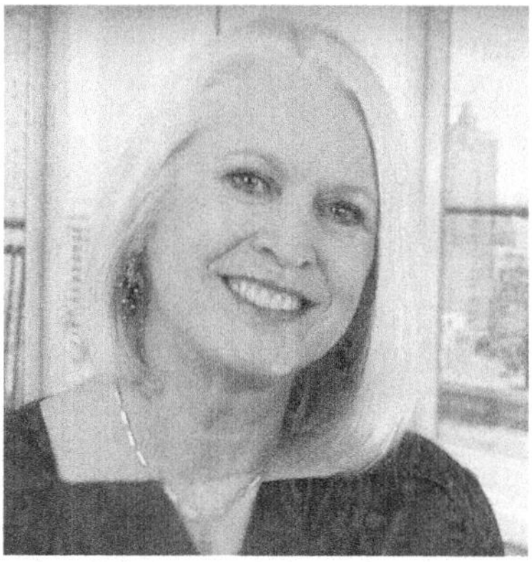

Paula Black's journey into health and healing began in one of the most difficult seasons of her life—a cancer diagnosis that threatened to take her life. Rather than accept it as the end of the story, she chose to seek deeper understanding—learning what cancer is, why she got it, and how she could restore her health.

What followed was a journey of faith, discovery, and transformation that touched every part of her life —body, soul, and spirit.

Today, Paula is an author, speaker, and faith-based wellness coach, helping others navigate their own healing journeys by blending the natural laws of health with the spiritual laws of faith and healing.

She walks alongside those facing cancer and other chronic health issues, offering encouragement, practical guidance, and a foundation rooted in God's truth. Her heart is to help people see that healing is possible—and there is a path forward. No one should walk a cancer battle alone.

Calling & Mission

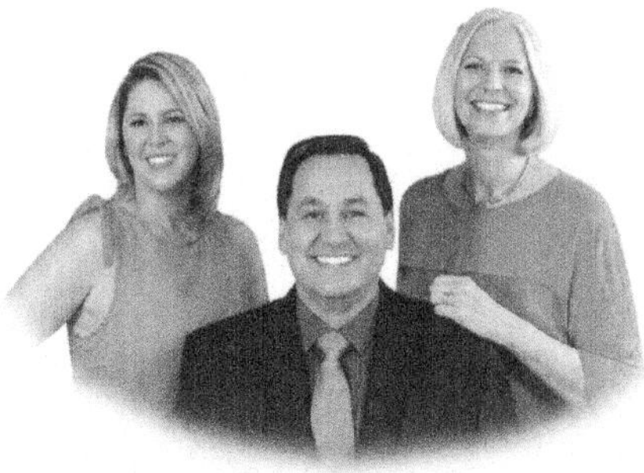

Dale, Paula & Kara Black

Our books at Black Eagle Publishing LLC, have a reputation for honesty, integrity, and spiritual clarity. We won't compromise the message, even when it costs us personally.

We've been banned, threatened, hobbled and defunded for refusing to compromise. The messages God has given us are possible because of the support of readers like you.

Join the mission and keep these messages coming.

JOIN THE MISSION
Help Change Lives

Visit **PaulaBlack.org** and "JOIN THE MISSION"

Before You Go...

Don't Miss Your…

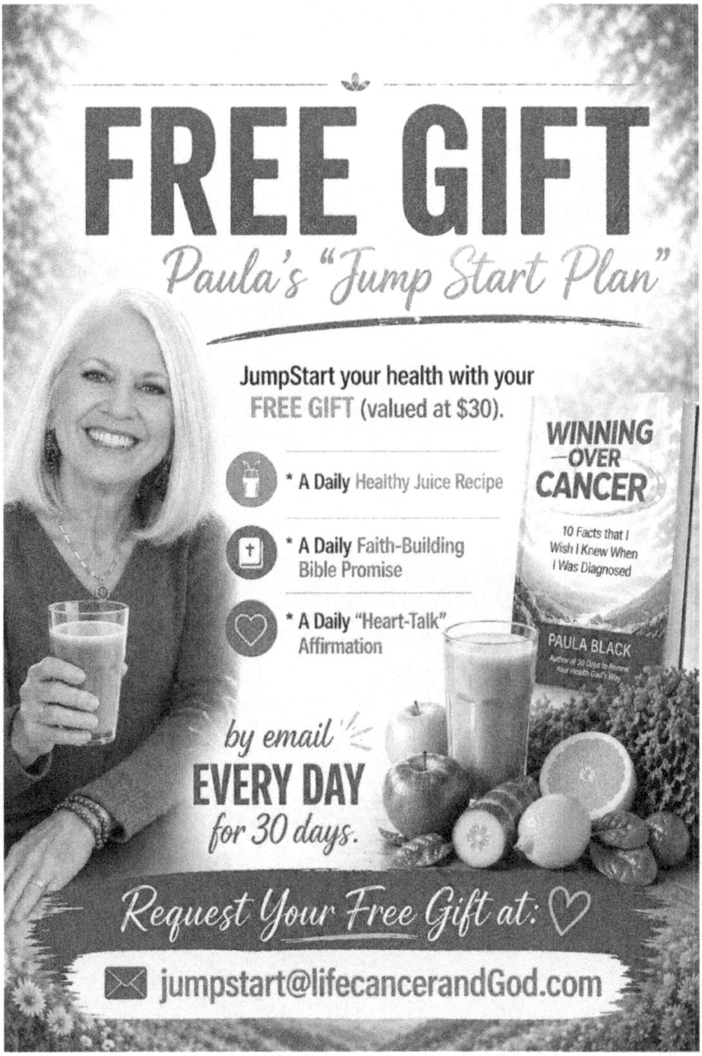

Someone Have Cancer?

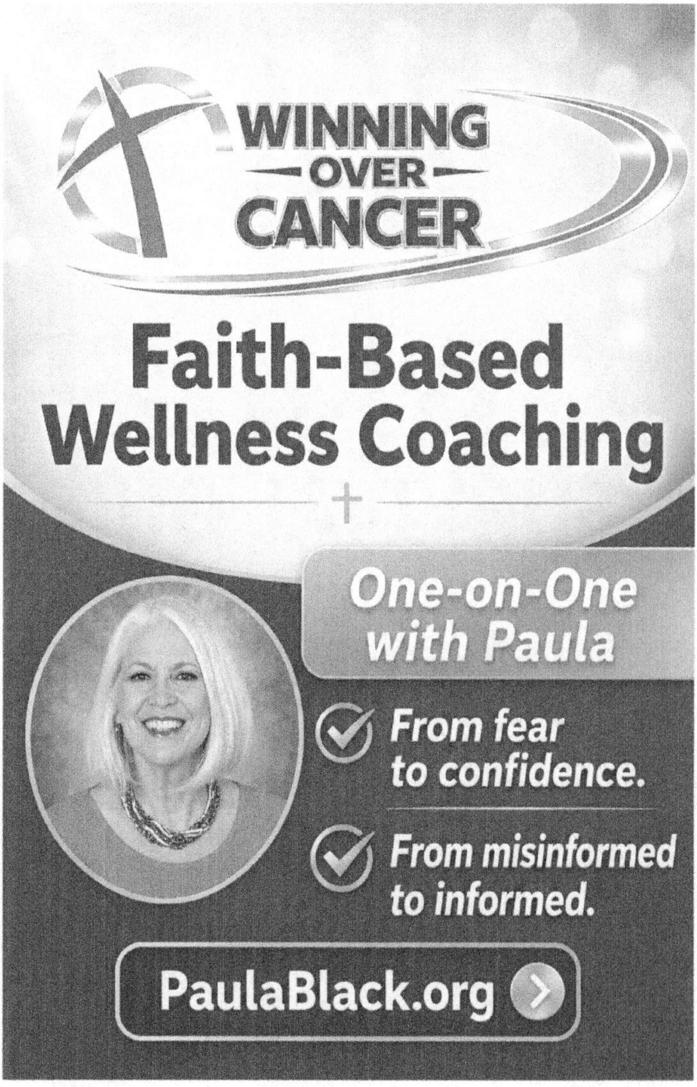

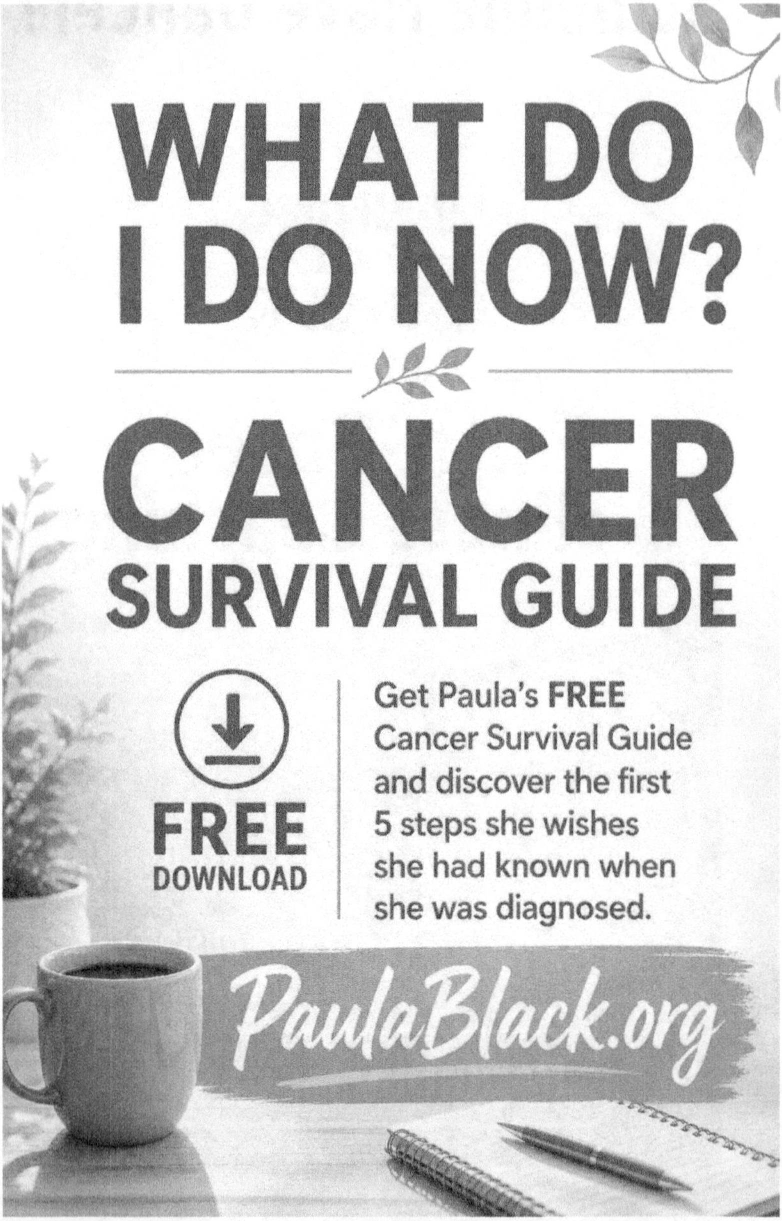
WHAT DO
I DO NOW?
CANCER
SURVIVAL GUIDE
FREE
DOWNLOAD
Get Paula's FREE
Cancer Survival Guide
and discover the first
5 steps she wishes
she had known when
she was diagnosed.
PaulaBlack.org

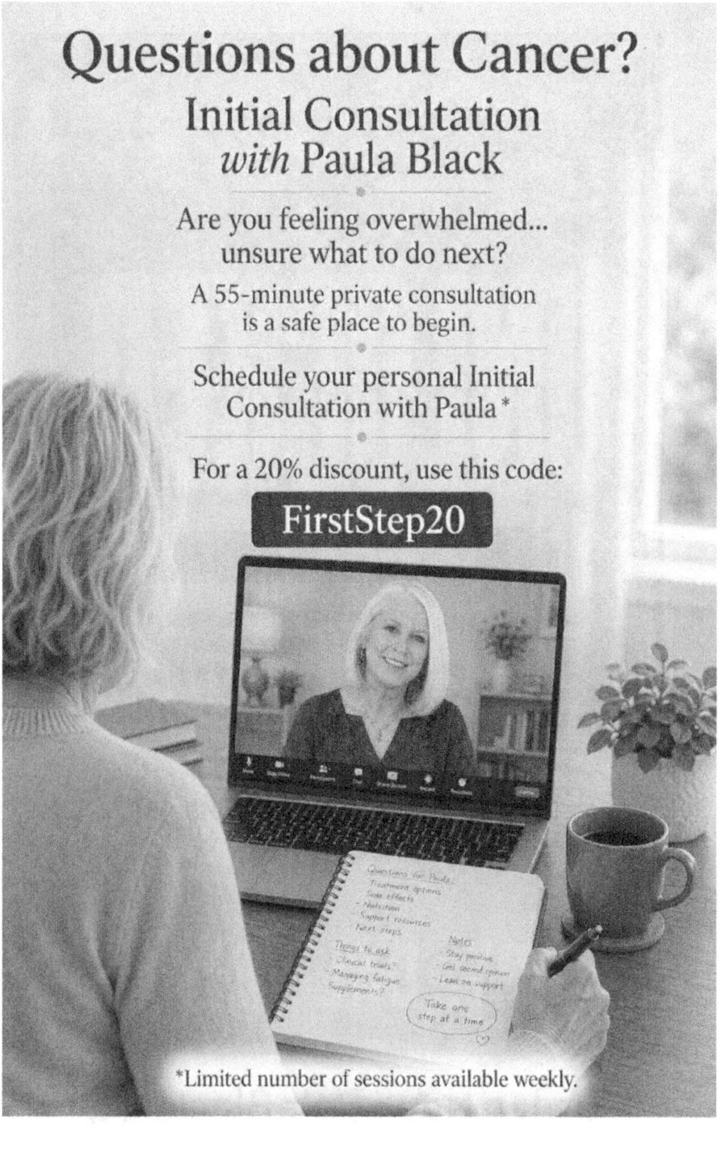
Questions about Cancer?
Initial Consultation
with Paula Black
Are you feeling overwhelmed...
unsure what to do next?
A 55-minute private consultation
is a safe place to begin.
Schedule your personal Initial
Consultation with Paula *
For a 20% discount, use this code:
FirstStep20
*Limited number of sessions available weekly.

The Shocking Truth About Cancer

Order Now: DaleBlack.org

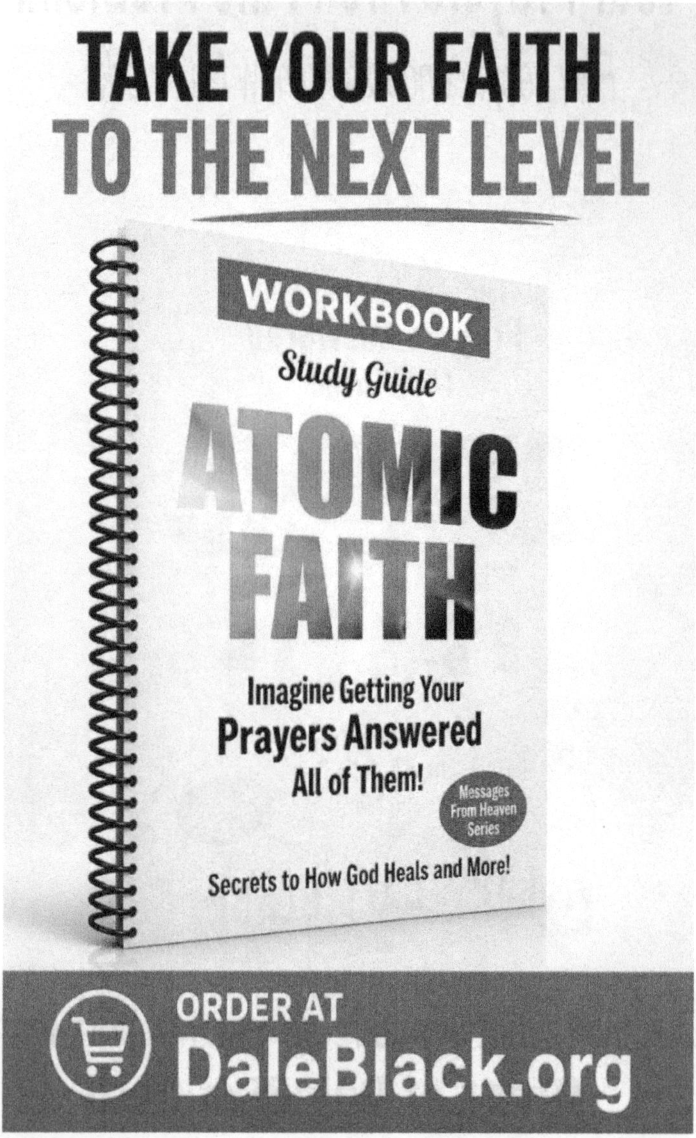
TAKE YOUR FAITH
TO THE NEXT LEVEL
WORKBOOK
Study Guide
ATOMIC
FAITH
Imagine Getting Your
Prayers Answered
All of Them!
Messages
From Heaven
Series
Secrets to How God Heals and More!
ORDER AT
DaleBlack.org

LIFE COACHING

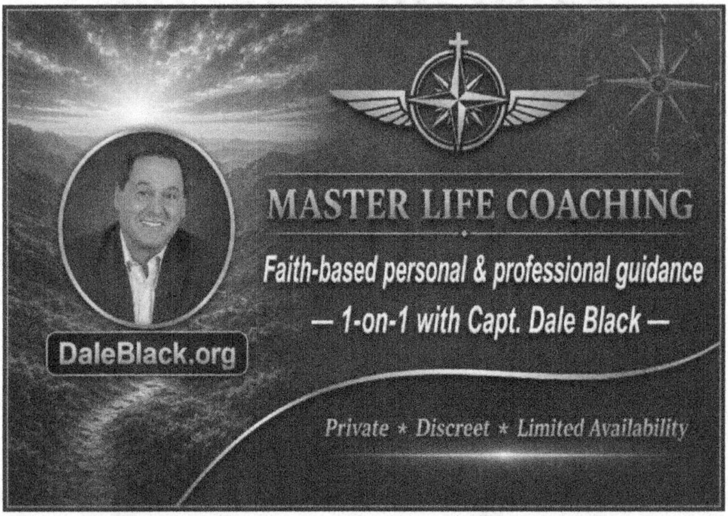

Discreet, faith-centered life coaching for individuals who value privacy, depth, and spiritual clarity.

Limited Availability

DaleBlack.org

Meet Jesus

No matter where you are in life...

whether you are full of faith,
full of questions, or
somewhere in between...

there is hope.

†

If you'd like to explore who Jesus is
and what it means to truly know Him,
I created a page just for you.

Visit

PaulaBlack.org

and click *Meet Jesus* in the top menu.

FOLLOW US

on Social Media

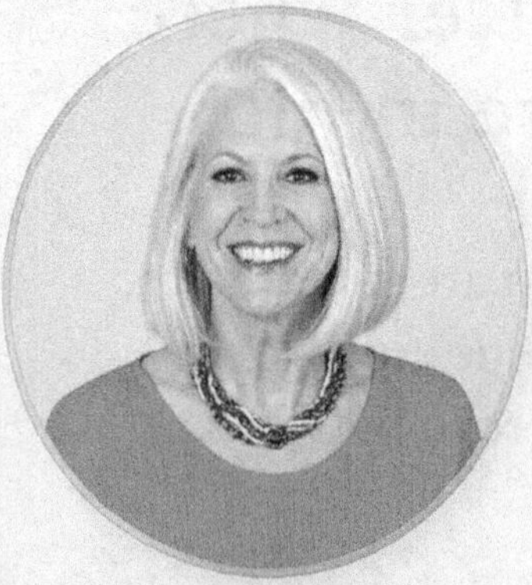

PAULA BLACK

PaulaBlack.org

@winningovercancer

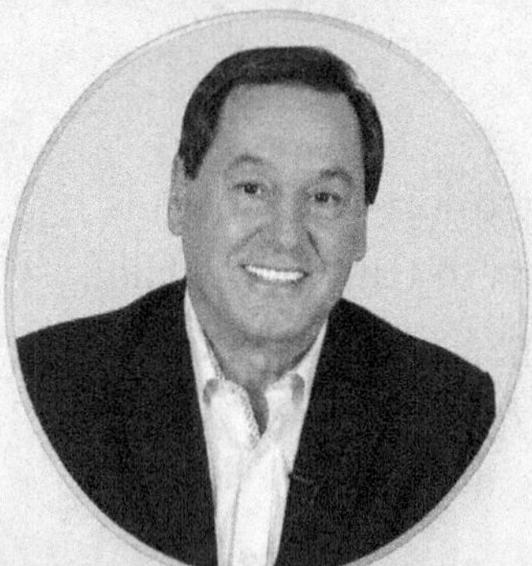

DALE BLACK

DaleBlack.org

@captdaleblack

Made in the USA
Monee, IL
13 September 2026

62980088R00104